D0042329

The Encyclopedia of

CONCENTRATED APHRODISIACS

The Encyclopedia of
CONCENTRATED APHRODISIACS

William H. Lee, R.Ph., Ph.D
and
Lynn Lee, C.N.

Instant Improvement, Inc.

The intent of this book is solely informational and is in no way meant to be taken as nutritional or medical prescription. Please consult a health professional should the need for one be indicated.

This book seeks only to tell people about substances that have been touted as stimulating to the sexual nature and not to suggest their use without the aid of a qualified health professional.

Instant Improvement, Inc.
210 East 86th Street
New York, New York 10028

Printed in the United States of America

Second Printing

Library of Congress Cataloging-in-Publication Data

Lee, William H.
The encyclopedia of concentrated aphrodisiacs / William H. Lee and Lynn Lee.
p. cm.
Includes bibliographical references (p. 327).
ISBN 0-941683-29-X
1. Aphrodisiacs--Encyclopedias. I. Lee, Lynn, CN. II. Title.
RM386.L43 1994
615'.766--dc20 94-28644

About The Authors

William H. Lee, Ph.D., is a registered pharmacist, nutritionist, and nutrition columnist for *American Druggist Magazine*. He is the author of many books and articles about nutritional subjects including, *New Power to Love, The Book of Raw Fruit and Vegetable Drinks, Concentrated Healing Foods*, etc. His articles appear regularly in *Health News and Review.*

Lynn Lee, CN (Certified Nutritionist) is Dr. Lee's wife and partner. She is an artist, art critic, author and lecturer. She has written and published *Anatomy of a Cold, Dream Control,* and a number of mystery stories, as well as co-authoring other books on nutrition.

Contents

PART ONE:

ENCYCLOPEDIA OF CONCENTRATED APHRODISIACS

C

F

G

M

N

O

P

W

X

Y

Z

PART TWO:

THE LOVER'S COOKBOOK

PART ONE

The Encyclopedia of Concentrated APHRODISIACS

Some Found Only
In The Dusky Confines
Of A Chinese Apothecary.
Some Found Among The
Leaves And Seeds In Your Garden.
Some Owe Their Reputation To Folklore.
Some Have Been Proven Effective At
Our Most Prestigious Universities.
All Are Revealed Here . . .

Preface

Fifteen years ago this book on Concentrated Aphrodisiacs just couldn't have been written.

All of us, of course, have heard of aphrodisiacs. And some of the wealthiest of us have, indeed, gained almost-miraculous returns to potency by being given one or more of them — often at $500 to $1,000 a treatment.

But it is only since the late 1970's that nutritional and medical science have discovered the revolutionary new techniques of compressing and condensing their active ingredients . . . making them far more powerful, and far more predictable, and at last costing only pennies per treatment.

Imagine what would happen if you took the most powerful aphrodisiacs in the world and concentrated them 10 to 100 times!

What is an aphrodisiac?

There are personal aphrodisiacs and general aphrodisiacs. Personal aphrodisiacs can turn you on but not necessarily anyone else.

Say, for example, that the first time you experienced that powerful thrusting power in your trousers, was when you kissed and were kissed back passionately by the female of your choice.

Say, you were both eating a chocolate bar previous to the simulating effect of libido.

From then on, the taste of chocolate, the smell of chocolate . . . even the thought of the dark, creamy, exotic feel of chocolate on your lips and face can stimulate your body into full sexual battle gear.

For you, chocolate is an aphrodisiac.

The power of an odor, a taste, a feel to stimulate memory is familiar to anybody for whom a whiff of perfume or cologne has automatically stirred lusty thoughts. It has even been proved in a research laboratory where college students who smelled chocolate during a word exercise and again the next day did better at remembering their answers than others denied the memory-evoking aroma.

The researcher, Frank Schab, said a memory strategy based on odor could help students studying for exams. His work provides the first firm scientific evidence that odors help bring back memories, said Brian Lyman of the Monell Chemical Senses Center in Philadelphia.

That may be the first scientific proof concerning odors and memory, but folklore has centuries of proof.

Baby powder, innocently applied to your genitals by a loving mother, the caress of a silken sponge, or — perhaps more destructive — a gentle slap on the rear end cause you didn't call for the "potty" — can be personal aphrodisiacs.

But these, and other "turn ons" like leather, spike heels, bondage, etc. can't be the subject of this book. The aphrodisiacs described here are universal. They have been tested by countless numbers of people who swear that their effects are true.

They work by influencing chemicals in the brain, or by stimulating hormones, by irritating sensitive tissue, by supplying needed nutrients, by concentrating themselves in the testicles, or by some mysterious means that only works for you.

Mostly it's men who search for an aphrodisiac. When faced with the vessel of love that can absorb many more strokes than they are capable of delivering, the thought of a source of additional power is as important as salvation itself.

Somewhere in this book is your answer. Somewhere among these pages is the trigger to "unendurable pleasure indefinitely prolonged."

Introduction

It should come as no surprise that roots, seeds and leaves have the power to heal. After all, a quarter of the more than $17.8 billion worth of drugs sold in the United States every year are derived from plants: birth control pills, aspirin, digitoxin, morphine, reserpine. So why should it be a surprise that herbal remedies and "old wives potions" should be effective stimulants to the reproductive process?

You may think that you don't believe in herbal and folklore remedies, but if you believe in ergotamine for migraine headaches and levodopa for Parkinson's disease, then it's just the packaging that has deceived you. We trust the synthetic nature of the sleek capsule or the pressed tablet but it is the grizzled bark, the crumbling leaves, and the earthy tubers that serve as the original source.

And all of them have undergone a couple of thousand years of clinical trials by being used by satisfied customers.

Not all remedies are plants.

The Chinese believe in the efficacy of dried sea horse. Its zoological name is *Hippocampus kelloggi*, and the Chinese call it Hai Ma. Dried sea horse, crushed and simmered in wine may not sound like the first course in an amorous adventure, but in China the concoction is traditionally used to "warm the kidneys" — for impotence. Something in the sea creature may indeed affect sexual hormones. A sea horse extract given to female mice prolonged the time they were in heat and increased the weight of the uterus and ovaries.

Where do the various substances people use for aphrodisiacal purposes get their reputation? Mostly through trial and error. What works is passed on from generation to generation and what fails is forgotten.

White Willow Bark

Sometimes there is a fable connected to a particular herb or substance. This one is about the use of White Willow bark. It is not an aphrodisiac but the story about its discovery is charming.

Back in the days when animals and humans could speak to each other and understand, a deal was made between King Beaver and the Indians of the American West. The Indians would kill only old beavers past their mating prime, and only as many as needed for warm clothes. One day, an Indian was suffering from a terrible headache. He was working on an old beaver he had killed but his headache was blinding him. In desperation he drank some water from a nearby shell not noticing that it held the genitals of the beaver he was preparing. To his great surprise and happiness, his headache disappeared almost at once.

When he tried to retrace his activities to try to understand his cure, he noticed the shell with the beaver's testicles. Later that day, as he related his story to the tribal elders, he mentioned the shell and the testicles. One of the elders had a terrible headache the next day and remembered the story. So he went and found a beaver and removed his testicles, soaked them in water, drank the water and recovered almost at once.

The story made the rounds of the various tribal meetings and, soon, beaver testicles were prescribed as a standard remedy for headaches, toothaches, fever, arthritis, rheumatism, and so on.

Before long, the low, gruff bark of the beaver was being replaced by a high shriek. King Beaver was very disturbed, so he went to the Indian Chief of Chiefs with a proposition. He would reveal the secret of the beaver testicle efficacy if the Indians would not mutilate any more beavers.

The Chief agreed and King Beaver took him to the White Willow tree. The bark of this tree contains the medicine to cure many things. When the beaver chops down the tree to build a dam, the medicine concentrates in his testicles. You can boil the bark and drink the resulting mixture for the same effect.

Since that day till now the deal made between the Chief and King Beaver has held true and Indians no longer slaughter beavers unnecessarily and no longer deprive them of their testicles.

Perhaps the story is not quite true in all of the details, but the White Willow bark contains salicin. Salicin was the inspiration for acetyl salicylic acid which we know of today as aspirin. The Indians did use it for the same reasons we use aspirin today and with the same results. Trial and error or King Beaver and the Indians . . . what's the difference as long as it does what folklore says it will!

Mandrake

The earliest mention of an aphrodisiac is in the Bible. It was not used to inspire lust but to escape the possibility of being barren.

In GENESIS XXX, v.14, 15, 16, 17:

And Reuben went in the days of wheat harvest, and found mandrakes in the field, and brought them to his mother Leah. Then Rachel said to Leah, give me, I pray you, of thy son's mandrakes.

And she said unto her, is it a small matter that you have taken away my husband? And wouldst thou take away my son's mandrake also? And Rachel said therefore he shall lie with thee tonight for thy son's mandrakes.

And Jacob came out of the field in the evening, and Leah went out to meet him, and said, Thou must come in unto me, for surely I have hired thee with my son's mandrakes and he lay with her that night.

And God hearkened unto Leah, and she conceived, and bare Jacob the fifth son.

In SOLOMON'S SONG:

The mandrakes give a smell, and at our gates are all manner of pleasant fruits, new and old, which I have laid up for thee, O my beloved.

What is known about the mandrakes from these and other passages in the Bible is that mandrakes were gathered during the wheat harvest and then, either for their rarity, flavor, or more probably their supposed quality of removing barrenness in women, as well as for their sexually-stimulating power, were greatly valued by the female sex.

The opinion respecting the peculiar property of mandrake was not confined to the Jews, but was entertained by the Greeks and Romans as well, the former of whom called its fruit *love apples* and bestowed the name Mandragoritis upon Venus the Goddess of Love.

Pythagoras was the first (followed by Plutarch) who gave this plant the name of mandrake (man-likeness). Dioscorides remarked that the root is to be used in love philtres, exciting the amorous potential, remedying female sterility, facilitating conception and — strangely — that female elephants after eating the leaves are seized with so irresistible a desire for copulation that they run eagerly in every direction in search of a male.

Speaking of the plant, the elder Pliny says it has a striking resemblance to the organs of generation of either sex. The male root, having arms and legs and a penis and being hairier than the female root, is a guarantee of amorous love with the woman of choice.

Strong warnings accompany this plant. It is said that the plant, upon being yanked from the ground, will emit a scream so piercing that anyone within hearing range will immediately go mad. Dogs were employed as "root pullers." A stout string was tied around the plant and fastened to a harness around the dog. The dog was then induced to run, thereby removing the root from the ground without causing harm to the root hunter.

How does the mandrake find its way into this world? The usual explanation is that it springs from beneath a gallows from the soil that has been moistened by human semen as a result of strangulation.

As Havelock Ellis and others have pointed out, strangulation frequently produces erection and ejaculation, and many a hanged man has ejaculated as he was hung.

In the fifteenth century, the mandrake enjoyed so great a reputation in Italy as an erotic stimulant that Machiavelli wrote a much admired comedy called La Mandragora.

It was also in the fifteenth century that the English parliament, summoned by King Richard III upon his usurping the throne, publicly urged, as a charge against Lady Grey, that she had bewitched King Edward IV by strange potions and amorous charms.

Mandrake had entered the royal palace!

What is this fantastic plant, how did it get its reputation and what does modern science say about it?

Mandragora officinarum — devil's testicle, mandragora, Satan's apple.

When witches brewed their magic potions, they seldom left out the mandrake root. It is a member of the potato family, along with other potent plants such as henbane, belladonna, datura, Jimson weed. It has a particularly high content of mandragorine (a powerful hypnotic and narcotic) as well as the alkaloids atropine, scopolamine, hyoscine and hyoscyamine.

This may be the grandaddy of the Mickey Finn. A wine brewed from an extract derived from boiling the crushed root can cause all sorts of trouble. Drink a little and anything goes. Drink a bit more and you're off on a big trip. Too much and you can fall into a deep trance ending in a three-day coma or even death.

How did the ancient peoples deal with the power of the mandrake without courting death? They used just a bit of the root — enough to escape their humdrum lives and release their libido. They knew enough of its power to respect it.

Some years ago, a book was written about the use of mandragora wine by the Romans for the victims who were being crucified. The book made a case that some of the crucified fell into a death-like coma, only to be revived days later.

Truth or fiction, it's another chapter in the story of a plant and the uses mankind has made of it.

We can't go into as much detail on the thousand or so herbs described in this book, it would take an encyclopedia many times its size. However, some plants will be dealt with at greater length than others.

Plants, including those we use for food, are only one aphrodisiacal area to be covered. Deer sperm, bird's nests, beetles and other substances will also be explored.

Instant Aphrodisia

Bubble, Bubble,
Toil and Trouble,
Cauldron Boil and Cauldron Bubble . . .

Forget it! This is the nineties and we have the blender to use in making our witch's brew.

Kava Kava

Piper methysticum

Found in most of the Pacific Islands from Hawaii to Polynesia and New Guinea.

- Also called ava ava or yangona.
- Part used: the roots of this shrub pepper plant.

Kava Kava has a history of religious and spiritual connections with mankind. This is one story of its part in the cycle of life and death.

Every year, a girl of wondrous beauty was offered as a sacrifice to the Sun. This one year, the greatest beauty ever found on the island was called Ui and she was chosen to be the Sun's bride. However, in this instance, the Sun was so pleased with her that he transported her to his side and took her as his wife.

After a time Ui became pregnant and asked to be returned to her people for the birth. The Sun consented and she flew through the air back to her birthplace. But, as she flew through a storm, she miscarried.

The fetus, being released in the air, fell into the water where it was found by a hermit crab who cared for the child and raised it. When the child, called Tagaloa Ui, reached maturity, he taught the Kava Kava ceremony to the people and insisted on the proper reverence. While the ceremony appears to be laughable to modern eyes, because the Kava Kava root is chewed and spit into a communal bowl and the saliva acts upon the root to release some of the active ingredient, it is considered sacred to those people who practice it. Pava, the first mortal to whom the Kava Kava ceremony was taught, had a son who laughed as his father chewed and spit. This angered Tagaloa Ui who cut him in two. When the brew was ready, however, Tagaloa Ui poured some of it on the son's head and made the boy whole again.

If you're in the islands and take part in the ceremony, you'll find that the root has a lilac odor but a soapy taste. The chewing is necessary to emulsify the active components in the root which are not water soluble but are made partly so by the action of saliva. Its taste is by no means delightful but you will never forget the first time you and your partner witness its effect. When it is brewed in water it makes a mildly stimulating tea. The tea can arouse a gently sleeping libido, but is not as aphrodisiac in nature as when it is prepared in other ways.

Chemistry of Kava Kava

The active constituents in Kava Kava are resinous alpha phyrones. They are soluble in alcohol, oil, and other fat solvents.

When the Kava Kava liquid is placed on the penis or the clitoris, the result is at first a mild tingling of the extensive nerve network in this extra-sensitive area and then a slow, ever-so-slow buildup of tension in the deepest musculature before an explosive mutual climax.

If you are an unfortunate sufferer of premature ejaculation and feel cheated of more sustained lovemaking, pat some of the Kava Kava oil on the head of your too-anxious organ. This will give you all the time in the world to finish what you started because the oil will allow you more relaxed control of your ejaculation and longer, more satisfying vaginal contact.

Kava Kava is available at many herbal stores but I can't see the average American Bar B-Q with a handful of invited guests sitting in a circle chewing on the root and spitting into a big bowl.

So, here's the modern method minus the philosophy, meditation and religious connotation:

Take one ounce of bark and chop it into small pieces or put it through a coffee grinder.

Place the Kava Kava in a blender and add two tablespoons of coconut oil (or any good food oil) and 1 tablespoon of lecithin granules or lecithin powder (also available at your herb shop or health food store).

Add one and one-half cups of water, coconut milk or skim milk and a handful of chopped ice.

Blend well.

Strain.

There's enough for four people and an orgy, or two people and a couple of tussles. If you have any left over, make ice cubes for later on.

The only problem is that you will get very sleepy within an hour after drinking the Kava Kava so be sure that your love object is close at hand. If you mix the potion, drink it and then have to pick up your date and the traffic is terrible . . . you'll find yourself amorously involved with the steering wheel!

But . . . there's more!

The active resins kawain ($C_{14}H_{14}O_3$), methysticin ($C_{15}H_{14}O_5$) and yangonin ($C_{15}H_{14}O_3$) can also be extracted by mixing with alcohol. Then, you can evaporate the alcohol in a double boiler leaving the resins behind.

Scrape up the resin and roll it into a number of pills. Then, when the occasion arises when another rise is anticipated, dissolve one of the small pills in warm brandy and sip.

And whoever said Kava Kava had to be applied to any bodily part by using your hands? Outside of a slight numbing effect, Kava Kava can also be placed on the tongue.

The Kava Kava alcohol extraction and subsequent mixing in warmed vodka or brandy is the most potent method, since the alcohol will carry the stimulants in minutes into the system, right where you need them. It will also make you sleepy.

When you buy Kava Kava, look for roots that are more than six years old. The bigger and thicker the root, the older it is. The root reaches a thickness of three to five inches in four years, and after six years it can weigh as much as twenty pounds. The most prized are those plants which have lived twenty years with roots weighing upwards of one hundred pounds.

Is there caution to be observed with this gift of Nature? Certainly! Constant and excessive use of the root and alcohol can become habit-forming. The skin can become yellow, the eyes can be bloodshot, and there can be a general loss of energy.

However, when the Kava Kava is discontinued the symptoms will usually disappear within a month.

Folklore is usually the basis for the use of certain substances. Now, however, these all-natural concentrated aphrodisiacs have been thoroughly tested and proven. They are now waiting for you — to give you the return to potency that even dangerous drugs could not promise you before.

Yohimbine

The next aphrodisiac has been tested and found to be authentic at some of our most prestigious universities. The aphrodisiac is derived from a tree called Corynanthe yohimbe and the substance is named Yohimbine.

The reddish brown inner bark of the tree has been available in the West since the 1930's when Norman Douglas called it the most effective of modern provocatives. It is one of the precious few potions that will excite a genuine undeniable sexual arousal within an hour, as opposed to a general tonic effect over a longer time span.

Stanford University called it a "true aphrodisiac."

Science Digest heralded it as "a cure for impotence."

Time magazine described it as "touted for years as an aphrodisiac."

Although the plaudits ring out in favor of the truth about yohimbine, the Food and Drug Administration continues to deny it.

In their Home & Garden section, the *Sun-Sentinel*, Friday, May 11, 1990, ran a long and comprehensive article about love drugs. Even in Florida, the home of the retired and the elderly, the thought of a workable aphrodisiac inspires a lot of interest. The article covered the Bantu tribe and its use of the bangala plant, American Indians and the use of Jimson weed, ginseng and so on. Most of the article was devoted to yohimbine and makes note of the FDA's regulation which prohibits marketing of any over-the-counter product which makes claims like: "improves sexual performance", "improves sexual desire", "helps restore sexual vigor", "builds virility and sexual potency."

Among the substances the FDA says are ineffective are: anise, fennel, ginseng, goldenseal, licorice, mandrake, nux vomica, sarsaparilla, vitamins and . . . yohimbine!

That has to make most people selling herbs a little wary. Even though Stanford University has shown it (yohimbine) to be a true aphrodisiac, if a store sells the herb as such it is subject to FDA action. In spite of the current research to make it available to the public, the FDA feels it has not been subjected to the extensive testing needed to formally establish it as "safe and effective." Mark Blumenthal, executive director of the American Botanical Council in Austin, Texas has called it a potent herb with at least the potential for abuse. Okay, so what about alcoholic beverages, pollution, antibiotics in meat, salmonella in chicken and eggs, etc? It's up to you. We present the facts, you make your decision.

In 1984, *Science* magazine carried the report about yohimbine and the Stanford endocrinologist Julian Davidson. It said that laboratory rats given yohimbine had increased sexual arousal. Not only did it increase the sexual activity of experienced males, but it induced sexual activity in previously inactive males (seems to cover about all of the males in the world!).

Yohimbine has centuries of use in Africa and the West Indies. In 1968, the first scientifically credible evaluation of its power was made by a Phoenix physician, Dr. W. W. Miller. He used a prescription drug called Afrodex which used yohimbine as its active component.

The results were, in the words of one participant, "quite spectacular."

Twenty-one patients took a placebo for four weeks, then Afrodex for four weeks. Another group of men took the same pills in reverse order. The test was a double blind one since neither group knew which pill was which.

Before the study, the patients in the first group reported three weak arousals a week and three climaxes. After four weeks on the placebo, they reported an increase to eleven erections and eight orgasms a week. This is due to the psychological effect that some placebos are able to generate by stimulating the body's own resources. However, after only a month on Afrodex, the same men reported a prodigious forty-nine full arousals and twenty-three climaxes in a similar one-week period.

What's more, the men in the second group had even better results.

That was in 1968.

Why didn't you hear about it?

Because America has been, and will be, very puritanical when it comes to sexual matters. Rape, murder, violence is reported on the nightly news but anything that may enhance sexual pleasure is buried in an obscure journal.

According to other research done by Doctors Alvaro Morales and David Surrige of Queen's University in Ontario, yohimbine recreates potency by producing a massive flow of blood directly to your sexual organ, thereby compelling it to rise. It also stiffens its muscles so they contribute more and more to your organ's firmness and rigidity. This means even the most ordinary stimulation can result in a full arousal. Veterinarians and livestock breeders have used their knowledge of this drug to stimulate lazy bulls and stallions. Make no mistake, this is a powerful natural drug. It penetrates the blood-brain barrier to produce an increase in the pulse, sweating, physical restlessness, urine retention and an elevation of blood pressure. It also causes a mild psychedelic effect by blocking the neurotransmitters acetylcholine and epinephrine when taken in doses above 50 milligrams. Some aphrodisia can be brought about from its inhibition of serotonin and monoamine oxidase (MAO).

CAUTION:

Yohimbine should not be taken with sedatives, antihistamines, amphetamines, diet pills, alcohol, cocoa, pineapple, bananas and any food rich in tyramine. If you have diabetes, hypoglycemia, liver trouble, heart disease, kidney disease, peripheral vascular disease . . . stay away from yohimbine.

The mental changes can include heightened empathy and an increased emotional response rather than an LSD-like trip.

Yohimbine contains numerous alkaloids: rauwolfine, ajmalcine, corynanthidine, quebrachine. The crude bark and an extract of the bark appear to have the same activity. When the extract is available it is usually in the form of a white powder which can be dissolved under the tongue, snorted, or put into capsules and swallowed.

Before this breakthrough, you would have to buy ten pounds of raw bark to get this power — now only the TNT ingredient remains. So you can hold the full strength concentrated aphrodisiac between your thumb and forefinger.

Why suddenly can we concentrate the power beyond belief? Because, until now, if the actual aphrodisiac was found only in the leaves of a 20-foot high tree, we could use only a few of those leaves in our preparation.

Now, however, we have the technology to strip the tree bare, pack all its leaves into a single vat, crush out the aphrodisiac, and condense its raw power into a tiny pill you can hold between your fingers.

You get nothing but pure aphrodisiac power! And you get more of it in one tiny pill than you could have gotten before in a full year's supply.

Many couples report an increase in skin sensitivity with yohimbine, so much so that the ecstasy of body melting into body is felt for the first time.

Yohimbine Cocktail

Now that you don't have to put a bone through your nose and take an ax to the tree to find out if yohimbine is for you, try this, using a small amount to test its compatibility:

> *First, get some of the powdered herb at your local herbery. Simmer two to three teaspoons of the powdered bark in a pint of water.*
>
> *As the solution cools, add 1,000 milligrams of vitamin C to the mixture.*
>
> *Add honey for flavor, and make sure your date is next to you and just as interested as you are.*
>
> *Sip a glassful.*

The reason you should add the vitamin C is to make a compound known as yohimbine ascorbate. It is less likely to have bad side effects. When yohimbine is combined with hydrochloric acid, yohimbine hydrochloride is formed, an adregenic blocking agent that can alter your mood in a negative manner. It is not recommended.

It's a good idea to check your condition with your doctor before using this herb. You may not be aware of good reasons to avoid its use, or you may be partial to aged cheese after sex and not know that you can't have aged cheese with yohimbine.

Herbalists look at their products differently. If the reputation as an aphrodisiac has passed the test of time, we generally tend to accept it as truth. Here's a few herbs that have earned a good reputation with conventional and aphrodisiac views:

Damiana

Turnera aphrodisiaca

- Parts Used — Leaves

Damiana has stimulating properties and has been used traditionally for nervousness, weakness and exhaustion. It has been used to increase the sperm count in males and to strengthen the ovaries in females. Damiana is also said to help balance hormones in females.

It has been used in cases of:

- Bronchitis
- Hormone imbalance
- Hot flashes
- Menopause

However, when asked about its ability to stimulate sexual impulses, an herbalist might suggest the following:

Take 1 ounce of damiana leaves
1 ounce of saw palmetto berries
Grind to a fine powder in a coffee grinder.
Fill some 00 capsules (very large capsules).
Take one capsule three times a day and watch your hopes and other things rise to your expectations.

Another herbalist could have a slightly different formula:

Take equal amounts of damiana leaves, muira-puama, kola nut, cocoa leaf and celery in a pot.
Pour boiling water over the mixture.
Let steep for ten minutes.
Strain, add honey to taste, sip a cup daily.

Still another formula suggests:

Take equal parts of damiana leaves, muira-puama, kola nuts, cocoa leaf and celery and put them into a jar.
Fill the jar with vodka.
Let stand for two weeks, shake daily.

After two weeks, strain and have a shot daily.

Or:

Soak 1 ounce of damiana leaves in a pint of vodka for five days.

Pour off the liquid, straining it through a conical coffee filter paper, and set it aside.

Soak the alcohol-drenched leaves in 4 ounces of spring water for another five days.

Heat the water extract to 160 degrees and add 1/2 cup of honey.

Combine the alcohol extract and the honey-water extract in a jar and let stand for one month.

A sediment will form as the mixture clarifies. Siphon off the clear liquid.

Take a glass or two of the liquid at night.

The above formulas illustrate the difference between what is accepted by the establishment for a particular herb or herbal combination and what is taught in folklore.

In Brazil, where the herbal tradition is strong, the natives consider damiana tea to be a nutritional tonic. The tea is used as a kidney strengthener and for a slow build-up of an aphrodisiac effect. They're inclined to be more patient in the warmer climes.

Mexicans and Brazilians consider damiana to be one of the better tonics for correcting male erectile difficulties. Damiana is related to the poison strychnine. There was a prescription drug, Andro-Medicone, which contained yohimbine and strychnine plus other ingredients. The poison was in the formula to help increase muscle contractibility. Although damiana is a relative of strychnine, it is much safer. Livestock breeders have used the herb as a stimulant to lazy studs and a Philadelphia physician, W. H. Myers, M.D. has said 15 to 30 drops of damiana extract daily for impotent patients has been successful in all cases. It seems, therefore, that we have arrived at a moment when return to full manhood is inevitable.

Damiana is not only for men. If the tea is taken before bedtime, women at first report highly colorful erotic dreams. But over a period of time, tea-drinking women report that they become progressively more sensitive and open to any kind of stimulation, oral, manual or penile, of the clitoris.

To make damiana tea, simply simmer two tablespoons of the dried herb in a large cup of hot water for about five minutes. Strain and sip. Limit the intake to one cup a day.

The ancient Aztecs knew of this herb and also used it as a tonic aphrodisiac and a cure for impotence, but along came the white man and the missionaries and they tried to wipe the plant out of existence. Fortunately, sex was stronger than the missionaries' message and damiana was not completely forgotten. On occasion, the plant nux vomica is mixed with damiana to heighten its effect. Nux vomica is a source of the aforementioned strychnine and is not a recommended herb.

There is reason for the mixture. Both strychnine and damianin (an active ingredient in damiana along with a green oil) stimulate the nerves and sexual organs. However, to repeat myself, damiana is much safer to use.

Louis T. Culling, in his *Manual of Sex Magic,* describes his sexual rejuvenation after only two weeks of damiana tea every evening. He called it an infectious aphrodisiac as well as a physical one since it made even standoffish people unusually friendly.

Too much of the damiana tea can be damaging to the liver so keep your intake down to when you need it and don't abuse Mother Nature.

Damiana tea can be hurtful but what can you do when an orgasm hurts?

Head-Pounding Sex—Indomethacin Can Help

Benign orgasmic cephalalgia is not an aphrodisiac (newly discovered), nor a new technique from the Kama Sutra, but a headache — a sex headache.

The old cliché about women, "not tonight, dear, I have a headache" has to be changed to, "not tonight dear, I don't want a headache."

And it happens more to men than women!

These headaches are cousins of the exercise-induced headache and involve excruciating head pain either before, during or just after orgasm.

Obviously, these circumstances are not very amusing to the people who suffer from this condition. However, the condition is treatable.

Benign orgasmic cephalalgia tends to respond well to indomethacin taken prior to sex.

In this case, indomethacin could be considered to be an aphrodisiac!

On the following pages is an alphabetical listing of people, places, and things having to do with sexual stimulation . . .

A

Absinthe

This delightful liqueur is made in France from the herb *Artemisia absinthium*. This is a bushy plant with small yellow flowers.

Absinthe is a green colored liquid prepared from the plant plus oil of aniseed, marjoram and other aromatic oils.

A little can make you a lover, a lot can drive you into the booby hatch . . . no fooling.

Artemisia is also called wormwood and was dedicated to the Greek goddess Diana, who was also called Artemis.

Abutilon indicum

Indian mallow

This plant's leaves, when made into a tea by steeping for ten minutes, are reputed to be aphrodisiac in action. They contain mucilage, tannin, and traces of asparagine.

Acacia arabica

Babul tree

The gum derived from the acacia tree, when fried in ghee, is used as a nutritive tonic and an aphrodisiac in cases of sexual debility. Some recipes add sugar and spices to the ghee.

Achilles Tatius

A writer who lived in Alexandria in the fourth century A.D. He is the author of Cleitophon and Leucippe, a love story which touches on a variety of ways to consummate a love union. Erotic fiction was considered to be aphrodisiacal in nature.

Acorus calamus

Sweet flag

Here is an herb with many uses. It is an aromatic appetizer and a dispeller of alimentary gas. The roots have a pleasant smell and can be very useful in curing stomach infections. American Indians have used the bactericidal action of the root for toothaches and colds, while East Indian mothers made them into a tea for baby colic.

In India, Iran and Arabia it is used to raise the libido. It also strengthens the memory. So if you have the urge and the ability but just forget what to do, one Indian recipe is as follows:

Take two ounces of the dried root
One dram of coriander
Half dram of black pepper
16 ounces of water
Mix all ingredients and boil down to 12 ounces.

On the other side of the world, the Cree Indians chew on a two-inch pencil-thick piece of root daily as a sexual nerve tonic. More than that can act as a psychedelic. The root contains alpha and beta asarone to alter consciousness in as little as a ten inch span of root.

Persians believed that an infusion of calamus increased sexual potency.

German sources claim sexual disturbances can be cured by drinking, for ten days, 1/4 liter of cider in which 20 grams of calamus has been steeped.

Adenanthera pavonia

Bead Tree

A decoction of the bark or new leaves acts as an aphrodisiac.

Adrenaline

Ephedrine

This prescription drug is said to have occasional aphrodisiac side effects since it is a stimulant of the sympathetic nervous system.

Naturally produced stimulants can be manufactured to order in the brain by using the amino acids L-phenylalanine or L-tyrosine. They stimulate the aggressive neurotransmitters which govern sexual conduct.

Aelus

A physician in Alexandria in the second century A.D. He recommended the flesh of the lizard as an aid to ensure virility. In Africa, the *lacerta scincus,* an amphibious lizard, was commonly used, ground into powder and sprinkled on food when a powerful aphrodisiac was needed.

An Arab recipe for potency consists of Chinese cubebs, cloves, cinnamon, Roumi opium, ginger, cardamom, white pepper, and mountain lizard. Mix the entire mess together, pound well, boil in olive oil, add frankincense and coriander seed, then mix the whole concoction with honey.

Take after supper and wash down with a glass of rosewater.

Some people get stimulated when holding a lizard in their hands. For this purpose, use a live lizard so the squirming action can produce amorous stimuli.

Affion

This was a Chinese preparation of which the chief ingredient was opium and the secondary ingredients were garlic and onions. Must have been quite potent since its erotic effects were often brutal and violent.

Agate

Like many other stones, the agate has the reputation for stimulating amorous activity.

Agnus castus

Also called the Chaste-tree or Abraham's balm, it was a tree whose leaves produced an aphrodisiac effect. It might have been some kind of thistle.

Albertus Magnus

Medieval occultist and philosopher who, in the course of his many works, offers numerous formulas for love potions. One of these is a combination of the brains of partridges calcined into a powder and mixed with red wine. (Sure, white wine goes with the brains of fish.)

Alchornea floribunda

This herb is native to the Belgian Congo where it is called *niando*. The root bark is dried and then mixed with food. The meal will cause an intoxication that is aphrodisiacal in nature to some but tends to cause violent action in others.

Sometimes the roots are macerated for several days in palm or banana wine. The result is a drink that is said to inflame the senses and stimulate lust.

This herb can be as habituating as Cannabis so beware!

Alcibiades

Famous Greek political leader of the fifth century B.C. He was so involved in love's pursuits that his coat of arms included Eros hurling lightning bolts.

Algolagnia

A term used for the two sexual perversions of masochism and sadism.

Allium cepa

Onion seeds are considered to be able to stimulate lust.

In early Rome, Martial advised eating onions to remedy an exhausted penis.

When one of the heroes of the *Perfumed Garden* is required to maintain an erection for thirty days in order to gain the girl of his dreams, he does so by drinking honey and onion juice.

Petronious recommends snails and onions as a penile-fortifying dish.

Allium porrum

Leeks have the same reputation as onions and may be used the same way.

Allium sativum

Garlic

The Ainu of Japan consider garlic a gift of the Gods.

In 1931, Dr. W. J. Robinson, M.D. wrote the book, *Treatment of Sexual Impotence in Men and Women*. He included the following about the erotic virtues of garlic:

"There is one spice or condiment of which I hesitate to speak because it is held in such contempt. I refer to garlic. There can be no question as to its pronounced aphrodisiac effect. In fact, it stands at the head of the list. But many of our Anglo-Saxons would prefer their impotence to the alternative of not having to eat garlic."

Almonds

An aphrodisiac preparation described by Nefzawi in *The Perfumed Garden* is as follows:

> *Take a glassful of thick honey.*
>
> *Eat twenty almonds and 100 grains of the pine tree before bedtime.*
>
> *Continue for three successive days, then indulge yourself at the forked gates of Heaven.*

Norman Douglas recommends a soup made the following way:

> *Mix powdered almonds with the yolk of eggs. Add to chicken stock and heat. As it is cooling, stir in cream.*

This soup has good aphrodisiac potential particularly if the subject is rundown.

Alpina galangal

The Arabs believe this plant's rhizomes have aphrodisiac qualities although Europeans use it as a carminative and stomachic.

Amanita Muscaria

A substance found in this mushroom produces hallucinations and also heightens sexual intensities, with corresponding heightening of sensory channels, olfactory and visual senses, and a kind of love intoxication.

At the same time it must be warned that this is a most dangerous substance and people have died under its influence. This is not to be used without medical supervision even if you think you know what you are doing.

Amaranthus polygamus

Prince's Feathers

Seeds, roots, and leaves are used in a 1 to 10 decoction for impotence.

Amaranthus spinosus

Spiny pigweed

The seeds are considered to assist in excretion, benefit the virility, and also brighten your intellect.

Amatory Cooking

Among foods and dishes that are reputed to have an effect on love are beef curry, onion soup, herring roe, cheese soup, eggs, chicken curry, fritters made with apples, pears and pineapples, herring, and oysters. (See Part Two)

Amatory Intensity

Ovid, late of Rome, described the intensity of kissing as a preliminary to more penetrating love in his *Amores*.

"I saw their frenzied kisses, linking tongue with tongue."

Other means of provoking erotic conditions are also described. These are virtually visual aphrodisiacs.

Ambergris

Once in a while, a long while, a fisherman will come across a grayish-white waxy lump of something floating in the water. Depending on how long it has been there, it will either have a fecal odor or a hyacinth smell.

It is whale's vomit!

Until people knew what it was, they thought it was almost anything. When it smelled of feces they thought it was the excrement of one of the sea Gods. They rubbed it in their skin, hair and beards and it made them more amorous. They smelled it and it made them dream of naked women. They ate it and it made their blood pulse with lust.

Once its powers were known, royalty demanded its share. It was mixed with the most precious oils and herbs. Arab and Turkish rulers poured the richest coffee over a few grains of ambergris.

Cardinal Richelieu thought that ambergris helped him father a son at age 85.

Madame duBarry ensnared King Louis XV with the odor of ambergris since she bathed in a decoction of perfume and ambergris daily.

According to Gary Seldin's book, *Aphrodisia,* an elaborate recipe incorporating ambergris was prescribed by a medieval doctor called Zacutus Lusitanus. The ingredients are listed but the amounts remained in the doctor's memory only.

Misce:

Bole tuccinum — clay with iron oxide
Musk — the dried penile secretions of the musk deer
Aloe's wood — resinous wood of Aquilaria agallocha
Red and yellow sanders — Petrocarpus santalinus
Sweet flag — Acorus calamus
Cinnamon
Rhubarb
Indian myrobalan
Absinthe — wormwood, artemisia
Ambergris

Lazare Rivière, in his *First Treatise on Man and His Essential Anatomy,* provides a more precise formula:

Misce:

Ambergris, 30 grains
Musk, 40 grains
Aloes, 90 grains
Grind together then cover with brandy.
Distill slowly in a bed of hot sand, filter and take 3 to 5 drops daily in a little orange-rose-cinnamon syrup.

Boswell states in *Dissertatio Inauguralis de Ambra,* that 3 grains of ambergris speeds up pulse rate, improves muscular strength and mental faculties, and disposes one to desire.

What's in this material?

- Ambrein — an alcohol
- Benzoic acid
- Cholesterol
- Plus a lot of junk the whale was glad to get rid of.

It's true that cholesterol, in spite of the bad press, is the precursor of a number of hormones manufactured in the body, so maybe it is an aphrodisiac.

But eating whale vomit?

It's enough to make you contemplate becoming a monk!

Amorous Inducements

According to Ovid they include a suntan, cleanliness, neat dress, brushed teeth, a good haircut and well-fitting sandals.

Anacardium occidentale

Cashew

The nuts or seeds, when roasted, are said to excite the faculties, especially memory. So if you chase a girl but forget why when you catch her, eat some roasted cashews and enjoy.

Anacyclus pyrethrum

This plant, also called Spanish pellitory, is used medicinally as an aphrodisiac.

Anaxarchus

A friend of Alexander the Great who had wine poured for him and his guests by beautiful, naked women. It began the cult of visual aphrodisia.

Anchovies

In Southern European countries, they have long been thought of as lust-provoking.

Anethum graveolens

Dill

Dill seed and herb were often used with other herbs in exotic love philtres and aphrodisiacs.

It perfects digestion and provokes bodily lust.

Angel Water

Popular in the eighteenth century in Portugal. Shake together a pint of orange flower water, a pint of rosewater, a half pint of myrtle water. Add 2/3's of distilled spirits of musk and 2/3's spirit of ambergris.

Drink a glass at night as you prepare for a love tussle.

Anthropophagous aphrodisiac

How far do you go in the search for amatory satisfaction?

Monstrous ingredients have been used throughout the ages and compounded into philtres and ointments to achieve erection. In the Middle Ages, a recipe for sexual stimulation included the putrefied flesh of a human corpse together with the testes of a man and an animal, the ovaries of a female plus pimento and alcohol.

Ugh!

Ants

A medieval aphrodisiac recipe utilized black ants. Oil was poured over the ants and then the mixture was put into a glass jar, ready for use.

Anvalli

In the Hindu erotic manual named the *Ananga-Ranga* is the following erotic recipe:

> *Take the outer shell of the anvalli nut and extract the oil and juice.*
> *Dry in the sun and then mix with the powder of the same nut.*
> *Mix with candied sugar, ghee and honey.*

Aphrodisiac Ointment

In Hindu erotology, a suggested ointment to be applied to the penis to delay orgasm and sustain an erection is made from:

> *Flowers of Nauclia cadamba*
> *Hog plum*
> *Eugenia jambreana*

Aphrodisin

A proprietary preparation prepared from yohimbine, aronacein, extract of miura puama and other ingredients.

Apium graveolens

Celery

According to *Potter's Cyclopedia,* the seed of the celery plant is an aphrodisiac.

In Haiti, celery is used according to this formula:

> *Steep 3 pieces of celery in scalding water and allow to macerate for 1/2 hour. Then, strain, add sugar and drink a glassful every 15 minutes.*

Apium petroselinum

Parsley

Traditionally considered an effective aid in aphrodisiac directions.

Arctium lappa

Burdock

The stalks of Burdock picked before the burrs come forth, stripped of the skin, salted and peppered and eaten raw, increase the seed and stir up lust.

Aristotelian Recipe

In the *Golden Cabinet of Secrets,* a work attributed to Aristotle by error, there is a recipe for a love philtre.

Misce:

> *Elecampane seed*
> *Vervain*
> *Mistletoe berries*
> *Dry them well and pound them in a mortar.*
> *Serve in a glass of wine to bend women to your pleasure.*

Arris

A Hindu technique for dominating women sexually is to take a piece of orris root and mix it with mango oil. Place in a hole in the trunk of the sisu tree for six months. Remove and apply to your lingam.

Artemisia abrotanum

Southernwood

The dried herb makes a fragrant tea if steeped only a minute or two. It has great repute among older people.

Artocarpus heter-phyllus

Jak fruit tree

The fruit of this tree is one of the largest, ranging in weight from 20 to 30 pounds each, with some varieties producing fruit weighing as much as 80 pounds. The nut-like seeds are roasted and are said to be nutritious with aphrodisiac action.

Asafetida

Devil's Dung

This plant grows mostly on the Iranian-Afghani plateau and could be called the coprophiliac's choice of aphrodisiac.

It has the odor of fresh feçes . . . but more so!

It earned the name Devil's Dung in the belief that Satan scattered his body over the earth to illustrate the dark side of the Doctrine of Signatures.

The Doctrine states that God has put all things on the earth that cure all man's ailments. He made these things to look like the part of the body that the substance was to be used for. Walnuts look like brains and are to be used for head ailments. Oysters look like testicles and add amatory strength. Plants that grow in water are to be used to strengthen the excretory system, and so on.

When the herb is fresh, the odor is so penetrating with a rotten sweetness that it reminds us of the secret desires behind civilization's mask.

It is sometimes burned as an incense, it is used in Worcestershire sauce. It is a stimulant tonic for the alimentary canal and used for flatulence, colic, dyspepsia, and constipation.

It also contains ferulic acid, a stimulant to the brain and to the muscles. It increases blood pressure a bit and creates a feeling of warmth without an actual rise in temperature.

If you are tempted to try this "aromatic" herb, boil an ounce in a pint of water to make an emulsion. One tablespoon is an average dose.

It is also available as a tincture, taken 1/2 to 1 teaspoon at a time.

However, to bypass the taste, find pills. Beware, though. Since the volatile oil is eliminated through the lungs, travel in buses or trains at your own risk. If you find it to be stimulating to your love life, make sure your partner partakes of the Devil's Dung at the same time.

Asparagus officinalis

As a food, asparagus is rich. It contains an abundance of aminosussinamic acid and asparagine which affects the genitourinary area. An infusion of the roots taken in the morning for several days is said to incite erection.

Asparagus helps to remove ammonia from the blood which helps to relieve fatigue. It also is a diuretic and promotes the removal of waste.

Madame de Pompadour made asparagus sticks for herself and visitors, adding nutmeg, lemon juice, and the yolks of eggs.

Avena satina

Oats

When there are troubles due to nocturnal emissions, over-sexual intercourse and the member no longer responds to mental commands:

> *Gather the fresh green plant in August and pound it to a pulp. Then, macerate it with 2 parts by weight of alcohol. Take 10 to 15 drops of the mixture 3 times a day in water.*

Avena sativa

Considered to be an effective aphrodisiac if it can be found.

Averrhoa carambola

It has been reported that this plant acts as a stimulant to the reproductive organs of both male and female. An infusion is made of the crushed seeds. It has an intoxicating effect but larger doses may induce abortion.

Avicennia species

Mangrove

This plant exudes a green, aromatic, bitter resin that is considered to be an aphrodisiac in the areas around the Indian ocean.

Alphabet for Sex

In his *Alphabet For Sex*, as quoted by Eugen Duhren (Iwan Bloch) in his *Neue Forschungen ueber den Marquis de Sade*:

"A large number of foods and sauces are held to result in a stimulation of flagging sexual appetites, and to be suitable for illuminating once again diminishing desire and ability.

Many people ascribe a beneficial influence to the eating of fish, oysters, crabs, caviar, mushrooms — especially the morel — and various kinds of cheese, notably the Parmesan."

The Brothel of Dervieux

The mesdames who ran the elegant brothels were absolutely obliged to realize the aphrodisiac importance of the *petit-souper* and they vied with each other in figuring out excellent menus designed to draw the attention of the semi-impotent gallants of the fashionable world.

During the revolution, the cuisine at the brothel of Dervieux became especially talked about. Before they lost their heads, nobles indulged their sexual tastes fueled by selected foods.

B

Bamboo shoots

Popular in China, these vegetables are considered to produce aphrodisiac reactions.

Bananas

Considered to have stimulating properties probably because the shape resembles the male organ.

Barbel

This fish, prepared with onions and garlic, helps to restore virility.

Basil

This aromatic herb that is used as a condiment has been reputed to be able to assist a flaccid member.

Baudelaire

Nineteenth century poet, Charles Baudelaire in his *Les Paradis Artificiels,* described erotic fantasies helped by numerous doses of hashish.

Bauhinia tomentosa

Commonly known as the orchid tree, this plant is admired in Florida for its showy flowers. The seeds may be roasted and eaten for their aphrodisiac action.

Albertus Magnus

Albertus Magnus, medieval philosopher and occultist, offered numerous formulas for love potions. Most of them were not particularly appetizing. The best of his recommendations had something to do with powdered brains of a partridge mixed with red wine.

From The Perfumed Garden:

Take a glassful of very thick honey, eat twenty almonds and one hundred grains of the pine tree before bedtime. Continue for three successive days.

Beans

St. Jerome forbade nuns to partake of beans because, *in partibus genitalibus titillationes producunt.*

In the middle ages monks were told to eat certain foods to eliminate carnal thoughts and actions. Also, many foods were prepared in special ways to produce anaphrodisiac effects.

Beefsteak

Havelock Ellis, the sexologist, regards beefsteak as "probably as powerful a sexual stimulant as any food."

Beets

Pliny the Elder, Roman encyclopedist, mentions beets, carrots and turnips as having aphrodisiac value in erotic dietary.

Belladonna

Atropa belladonna

A dangerous herb which can yield a poisonous drug. Both the roots or the leaves contain alkaloids which, if concentrated, can give you the worst trip of your life . . . if you live. Atropine, hyoscine, belladonnine, hyoscyamine are found in the Deadly Nightshade.

Better impotent than dead!

Betel

Want to spend an ideal summer vacation—easy-to-wear minimum clothing, games, talk, climbing palm trees to gather fragrant orange-colored fruit and then amour in the tall grass?

That's the life of the gatherers of *pinang* in Malaysia, of *supari* in India, which we call areca or betel nut, and which is one of the world's most popular stimulants.

The orange fruit conceals brown seeds that are dried in the sun, then mixed with several other ingredients to make a wad that can be chewed on or sucked for hours. The result is a feeling of energy, euphoria, and sensuality that asks for a day and night of love.

The wad is made from a thin slice of areca, burnt lime (hydrated calcium oxide), and a sprinkle of catachu gum. The combination acts to release the alkaloids present in areca, arecoline — arecaine — guracine — arecaidine — central nervous system stimulants which increase the efficiency of the heart's pumping action.

Most of the users flavor the mixture with nutmeg or clove, wrap the whole mess in a leaf from the betel pepper plant and look forward to a day and night of uninterrupted fantasy. Betel leaf itself is a mild stimulant, saliva promotor and breath sweetener . . . which is handy considering the prospective lovemaking.

Is there a negative to this use of betel?

Sure! You can get dizzy, nauseous, diarrheal, maybe even convulsive. Your teeth will eventually be stained reddish-black and you will be spitting constantly. Now, red-black spittle may not be discouraging to the forest, but your living room and bedroom may not profit from the color scheme. Also, overuse will usually cause underuse of your "Mr. Happy."

Still, once in a while if you shop in an Indian grocery store, spit red and enjoy yourself.

Bhang

A Sanskrit term meaning hemp.

The leaves and seeds are chewed as a means of increasing sexual capacity.

The following formula is recommended:

Misce:

Hemp seeds
Musk

Sugar
Ambergris

The seed capsules and leaves can be made into an infusion with alcohol and then enjoyed as a liquor.

Bhuya-Kokall

Hindu plant named Solanum jacquini that has been suggested as an aphrodisiac by the *Ananga-Ranga* when made as follows:

Take the juice of the plant and dry it in the sun.
Mix with honey, ghee, and candied sugar.

Bird Nest Soup

The nests used are those of the sea swallow. The bird begins to build its nest with seaweed which dries in the sun. The leaves are stuck together with the bird's spittle and fish spawn which is loaded with phosphorus. Phosphorus is the one mineral you need for sex! You need it for desire and erection. Without it . . . give up.

The soup, when prepared correctly, is also heavily spiced. Many people swear by this concoction but have it made in a good restaurant or else you'll end up with a robin's nest and get nothing but diarrhea.

Birthwort

The early Romans thought of this herb as an aphrodisiac and it was used until the fifteenth century as such.

Bois Bande

A concoction called tightening wood that is used by the women in the West Indies. It is reputed to be an aphrodisiac. The main ingredient is the bark of a tree which contains brucine and strychnine. They will cause muscle toning but if the formula is prepared wrongly it can be a poison.

Borax

In the seventeenth century, borax was considered to be able to create powerful desires. Use with caution.

Brains

Calf, sheep or pig brains served fresh will act as sexual stimulants.

Brya

Pliny the Elder considered the ashes of the plant, when mixed with the urine of an ox, to be aphrodisiac.

Bufotenin

This substance is chemically related to mescaline. It is obtained from the venom of a particular toad and is also present in the seeds of the mimosa plant.

South American tribes use this an aphrodisiac in the form of a snuff called cohoba.

Although bufotenin does induce hallucinations of a psycho-erotic nature, its use is highly dangerous and it is not to be used without a guide or a physician standing by.

Burra gokhru

Seeds and leaves of this plant, used in India as a soothing diuretic for genitourinary infections, can also be used against impotence.

Officially named *Pedalium murex,* it can be utilized as follows:

Crush one part of seeds to twenty parts of water by weight.
Let steep for 24 hours.
Strain and add 1 ounce of vodka as a preservative.
Take one teaspoon three times a day.

This plant, while little studied in the U.S. may be almost as stimulating to the genital ganglia as yohimbine.

Madame duBarry's Table

Madame duBarry's table was laden with ginger omelettes, turtle soup, sweetbreads, shrimp and celery soup to spark the royal scepter.

Brillat-Savarin

The celebrated author Brillat-Savarin (*Physiology of Taste*) points out the importance of fish followed by the truffle:

"The tubercle is not only delicious to the taste, but it excites a power, the exercise of which is accompanied by the most delicious pleasures. The truffle is a positive aphrodisiac . . . it makes women more amiable and men more amorous."

C

Camel Fat

If one takes some fat from the hump of a virile camel and melts it down it becomes an aphrodisiac.

Cannabis indica

Indian Hemp

This drug has been used for centuries as an aphrodisiac. It grows in Central and Western Asia, in India, Africa and North America.

The resin extracted from the plant is called *cannabinon,* from which cannabinol stems, a red, oily substance found in the flowering tops of the female plant. Extracted from the plant in pure form, it is known in India as *charas.*

The powdered and sifted form of this resin is called hashish. A weaker form is called bhang and it is called marijuana in Mexico and the United States.

This plant has been known and used for 5,000 years in China. In 800 B.C. it was introduced to India. The Assyrians used it as a narcotic. Under the name Ma Fu Shuan it was used as an anaesthetic.

Cantharides

A species of beetle known as Lytta vesicatoria or mylabris, found in Southern Europe. It was known to Dioscorides, an army physician of the first century A.D. The active ingredient is a white powder prepared from the body of the bug. The powder used externally can cause blistering to the skin, taken internally it can be fatal. This fact did not stop the use of cantharides because the irritation it caused in the genitourinary tract was a stimulant to some people. In the eighteenth century it was mixed with flour to make cakes and bread and also mixed in candies and chocolates. The unwary guest would get a dose of cantharides whether they wanted it or not.

The beetle was and is a beautiful bug about an inch long with a head shaped like a valentine and with shiny gold and green colors. It's called Spanish fly and the Chinese have prepared a formula which includes saffron, syrup of honey, nutmeg, cinnamon, cloves and cubeb pepper. In India it's mixed with datura and can be an overwhelming experience despite the obvious danger.

Medieval Arabia and Europe had their own formula. In the *Geneanthropeia* of Sinibaldis is this cutie:

Misce:

Tincture of Spanish Fly, 1/2 teaspoon
Spanish lavender, 2 tablespoons
Spirits of Chloroform, 1 teaspoon
Water, enough to make, 8 ounces
Take 2 tablespoons 3 times a day.

Although its reputation exceeds its ability, people still believe in it. However, great pain or death can take the fun out of any seduction using cantharides, especially if both parties are not aware that even the tiniest dose can be dangerous.

Caperberry

In the Bible, the term caperberry is used synonymously with sexual desire. The berry was considered to be a sexual stimulant.

Capsicum annum

Paprika comes from this plant and Hungarians consider food made with paprika to be strongly aphrodisiac.

Caraway

Oriental love manuals frequently include caraway seeds in their love potions.

Cardamom

In Arab countries, the following dish is thought to promote erotic vigor.

Mix cardamon, ginger and cinnamon and sprinkle over boiled onions and green peas. Add a hardboiled egg or two and go on a picnic.

Carpolobia alba

This is an African tree with sweet edible fruit. The roots of the tree are regarded as sexually stimulating by the natives of South Nigeria.

Carrots

Stew carrots in milk sauce as a help in sexual activity.

Catancy

The witches of ancient Thessaly in Greece used the leaves of this plant as one of the ingredients in love philtres.

Catha edulis

Khat, Quat, Gat

The leaves have been chewed for centuries for their invigorating and sexually stimulating effects. It is also prepared as a tea.

The active ingredient appears to be norpseudoephredine and related alkaloids similar in action to amphetamine. It appears to be habit forming and is banned in some countries.

Chocolate

Anne of Austria brought chocolate to France when she married Louis XIII. However, it was not to become a rage until Louis XIV married the Spanish Infanta, Maria Theresa, who was a chocolate addict.

Casanova and duBarry considered it to be a love stimulant.

Brillat-Savarin searched for chocolate that was "sweet but not insipid, strong but not bitter, aromatic but not sickly, thick but free from sediment."

This incomparable gourmet experimented with chocolate mixed with pepper, allspice, aniseed, ginger, musk, orange flowers, rosewater, and other herbs but it was not until the introduction of vanilla and sugar that chocolate came of age.

The first solid chocolate was born in 1847 and the first milk chocolate in 1876 in Vevey, Switzerland by Daniel Peter and Henri Nestlé.

Why can hot, spicy foods be exciting?

British researchers at Oxford Polytechnic found that adding only three grams of hot chili sauce and the same amount of ordinary yellow mustard (three-fifth's of a teaspoonful) caused an increase in the metabolic rate of twenty-five percent on average.

That's twenty-five percent more of an inclination to do something after dinner instead of sitting on the sofa watching TV.

Add more of the spices than three-fifth's of a teaspoon and you may be able to shake the earth!

Caviar

Generally considered to be a sexual stimulant. In 100 grams of caviar there are 335 milligrams of bioactive phosphorus ready for metabolic activity. Caviar is the treatment of choice in cases of nutritionally reversible impotence, according to Dr. William J. Robinson in his book, *America's Sex and Marriage Problems*.

Celery

Want to whet your amorous appetite? Make a meal of celery soup. Both of you should eat of it.

Chameleon

Avicenna recommends the milk of chameleon as a sexual stimulant.

Cherries

Mentioned often as a stimulant when included in love cookery.

Chestnuts

Soak them in muscatel, then boil them along with satyrion, pistachio nuts, pine kernels, cubebs, cinnamon, rocket seed and sugar.

This recipe comes from an old English book on love philtres.

Chicken Eggs

W. J. Robinson, M.D., an authority on sexual impotence, said he often asked his patients to eat anywhere from 2 to 6 raw eggs first thing in the morning.

Egg nog is very popular in folklore to increase virility. Here's one recipe:

Take two eggs, 2 tablespoons of powdered sugar, 1/2 pint of milk, 1/2 pint of sweet cream, 6 tablespoons of brandy or whiskey. Beat egg yolks and sugar together until very light. Stir in milk and cream, then add brandy. Lastly, whip in the whites of the eggs which have been beaten into a froth.

This is another aphrodisiac mixture using eggs:

Fill a glass with the yolk of a fresh egg, 1/3 brandy, 1/3 maraschino, 1/3 creme de rose.

Chick Embryo

Daily doses of one seven-to-nine-day-old chick embryo is the prescription of some nutritional rejuvenating centers. The diet is said to restore all of the sexual functions to that of a teenager.

Chickpeas

Take the juice of powdered onions and add some honey. Heat until the onion juice is driven off. Then cool the residue and mix with water and pounded chickpeas. Take this before bedtime for an especially stimulating adventure.

Chocolate

Was once considered to be the most effective aphrodisiac by the American Indians. Even recommended by Havelock Ellis.

The Mayans mixed unsweetened, ground, roasted cocoa beans with corn beer.

Montezuma drank it mixed with snow from the mountains.

Linnaeus named it *Theobroma,* food of the Gods. And, the beans were so esteemed that they were used as money.

Cortes and his people came across cocoa in the Aztec capital of Tenochtitlan. But this was a different brew. He sampled *xoxo-atl,* a delicious, foamy beverage mixed with honey and flavored with thilxochitl (vanilla). This was the aphrodisiac consumed at rites dedicated to Xochiquetzal, the Aztec goddess of love.

When it was introduced to Europe it swept the land, was condemned by priests, and enjoyed by the masses.

Like all beans, cocoa has a fair share of protein, plus calcium, potassium, iron, and the mineral essential to erections — potassium.

Phosphorus, sugar, theobromine and the unique taste of cocoa can put you in the mood for love but there's more!

The moods we associate with romantic love are accompanied by a biochemical reaction resulting from the presence of a neurochemical called phenylethylamine (PEA). When there's a lot of this neurotransmitter racing around the brain, people experience a "high" similar to the feeling of being in love. Chocolate stimulates the production of that neurotransmitter and you, or whomever you share it with, will feel that "high" as though you both were in love.

Therefore, chocolate is the food of love, either as that bar of creamy delight eaten from sticky hands or other parts of the body or sipped as cocoa with whipped cream just before you hop into bed.

Chutney

A relish made of herbs, fruits and spices. It has a reputation for stimulating the libido.

Cinchona

Bark of a Peruvian tree. Contains alkaloids that have been used as a treatment for malaria. Previous to that, the bitter principle of the bark was said to inflame the senses.

Civet

Perfume derived from the civet cat. The secretions from the penile and anal areas of the cat formed the basis for perfumed chocolates which were eaten to stimulate desire.

Clams

According to the Law of Similars, because they look like testicles, as do oysters, they will stimulate desire.

Cola

Cola Nitida (also called *Kola)*

This was, at one time, the ingredient in Coca Cola after it became illegal to use cocaine in it! Today, though, even kola nut is not allowed in the great "American Drink."

It still is an extensively used refreshing drink in Jamaica and Brazil, its primary attribute being that it is a sexual stimulant similar in power to cocaine. The powdered seeds are used as a condiment by the natives of Africa, West Indies and Brazil. A small piece of seed is chewed to help digestion and it is said to improve the flavor of any food.

Its chemistry shows that it contains caffeine, theobromine and kolanin. It is a CNS stimulant, especially to the cerebral cortex and the medulla. It is a strong stimulant and economizes muscular and nervous energies.

You can try one tablespoon of kola powder in a cup of black coffee but add some honey to cut the chalky taste.

Cola

The flavoring of many soft drinks is derived from seeds contained within the pods of the tropical African cola tree. The seeds contain more caffeine than coffee, as well as some theobromine, and are sometimes chewed by West African people to allay hunger and ward off fatigue. A native cola drink is made by boiling the pulverized seeds in water for several minutes.

Colewart

The Romans dedicated this herb to Priapus and associated its use with lascivious activities.

Coriander

Albertus Magnus states that coriander, valerian and violet are love-producing herbs, but they must be gathered in the last quarter of the moon.

Cotton Root

Gossypium herbaceum

A decoction is made from the inner bark which contains an active resin. It is recommended for lust resurgence if interest in the opposite sex has waned.

Cow Wheat

Melampryum pratense

Although this tall plant with yellow flowers was used as a food for cattle, Pliny the Elder held that it inflames the amatory passions.

Crayfish

All seafood is considered to be of help to the sexual appetite. The crayfish, boiled in oil, with pepper, salt, garlic and other spices, can contribute mightily to a night of romance.

Crocodile Tail

The tail of young crocodile is considered to be a sexual delicacy.

The Roman poet Horace states that the excrement of the crocodile has aphrodisiac virtues.

(Perhaps he was referring to its effect on other crocodiles.)

Cubeb

Piper cubeba

The cubeb, indigenous to Java, is a berry similar to pepper with a more pungent flavor.

The Arabs and the Chinese considered cubeb to be strongly aphrodisiac in nature and prepared drinks mixed with honey as a sexual inducement.

Cumin

An aromatic plant used as a condiment and often assumed to have erotic stimulatory effects.

Cuttlefish

Cuttlefish, spiced oysters, sea hedgehogs and lobsters were among the ingredients of love potions used in the second century A.D. by Apuleius.

Cyclamen

The root of this plant was used in ancient times as a stimulant.

Cymbopogon schoenanthus

Camel Grass

The internal portion of the rhizome is considered to have restimulating power.

Cyperus esculentus

Earth Nut

Boil the nut in chicken broth, peel, add pepper and butter. This food is said to help older men perform like young men.

D

Darnel

A grassy herb that has a reputation for being a sexual stimulant to women if combined with myrrh, frankincense and barley.

Davenport

John Davenport wrote two essays dealing with sexual conditions: *Aphrodisiacs and Anti-Aphrodisiacs,* and *Curiositates Exotica Physiologiae.*

Deer Sperm

An example of organotherapy (the consumption of the genitalia of animals as a means of regaining sexual potency). The sperm was used as an ingredient in an aphrodisiac concoction.

Diasatyrion

In the brothels of old Persia, a drink was prepared to strengthen the penis. It consisted of satyrion and cow's milk and wine. It was said that seven days and nights of drinking this potion will transform old men into young men and make sure a man could enjoy everything — but everything — he was paying for.

Dionysus

Ancient god of wine and fertility. The phallus was ever present in the Dionysiac cult. In Lesbos, the god was worshipped as Dionysus Phallen. On the island of Rhodes a phallic festival, the Phallophoria, was celebrated with orgies.

Dita Seeds

Need help to maintain a hard-as-steel erection and prevent premature ejaculation?

This is the remedy used from India to the Phillipines. While the bark has been used as a remedy for painful menses, the seeds contain a substance called chlorogen ($C_{21}H_{20}N_2O_4$), reportedly a powerful aphrodisiac for men. Start with a tiny dose of less than 2 grams. Crush the seeds and let them stand in water for 12 hours. Then strain and drink the liquid and you have a hard-as-steel nightcap.

Dendrobium macrael

Indian Orchid

The plant, root and stem are made into a decoction to treat sexual debility in India.

Dog-Stones

A species of the plant satyrion (Orchis mascula) that had aphrodisiac properties.

Dove

Dove's brains, prepared in a mustard and dill sauce by master chefs were said to stimulate sexual desire.

Drepang

Also called Tripang. It is a Malay term for a species of holothuria or sea slug living in Oceans and in the Red Sea. The Chinese and Arabs consider it to be aphrodisiac in activity possibly because when it is touched it expands, much like the penis.

du Barry

Among the recipes she used to cultivate amorous action were ginger omelettes, stuffed capon, turtle soup, sweetbreads, shrimp soup, and crawfish.

Dudaim

The Biblical term for mandrake. (See "Mandrake", page 35)

Durio zibethinus

Durian

This large, spiny fruit of the Durio tree has been written about by many botanists and naturalists because it smells like rotten gorgonzola cheese to some, like dirty socks soaked in turpentine to others, and like custard that has been dragged through a sewer to still others. However, they all agree that once you have gotten past the odor, the taste is out of this world.

The tree is found in Indonesia, particularly in Sumatra, the Celebes and the Moluccas, and in Borneo, and everywhere it grows, the odor and flavor attracts every living thing from humans to animals to insects. It is profoundly aphrodisiacal and, since the fruit decays rapidly, the natives camp out near the trees during the fruiting season in order to be on hand as they ripen.

Madame de Pompadour

In the eighteenth century, Madame de Pompadour served Louis XV "hot" foods like fish, truffles, asparagus, vanilla and chocolate.

Being a King Is Not All That Easy

King Farouk of Egypt (1920–1965) created an image of being an insatiable lover, but in reality he had a low sex drive. He began each day with a banquet of not only eggs, but countless dishes of meat and fish. Unwise, since it contributed to his girth. Even though he was six feet tall, 300 pounds is a lot to carry around. Because he began to have bouts of impotence at age 23, he consulted hormone specialists, tried hashish mixed with honey and powdered rhinoceros horn. That, plus his diet, must have worked because he attempted sexual intercourse with approximately 5,000 women.

Toward a Longer, Sexier Life

Sexual exercise is a powerful life extender. According to *Sports Medicine* 1990;9:330-43, studies indicated a strong relationship between sexual activity and longevity.

As Masters and Johnson have pointed out, there is a strong parallel between the orgasmic response and exercise. So foods which help promote sexual congress may keep you living longer and happier than a severely restricted diet.

E

Echinops echinatus

Globe thistle

All parts of this plant can be used to prepare a decoction for seminal debility and/or impotence.

Eels

Like the rest of life found in the sea, eels are said to be aphrodisiac in nature. Eel soup is specially prized as such with spices, garlic and onions.

Eggs

The egg, the beginning of you and me, aphrodisiac in action since the days of old.

Duck eggs, raw . . . scrambled with truffles.
Chicken eggs scrambled with avocado.
Raw eggs mixed with brandy.

Or this recipe from *Venus in the Kitchen.*

Beat 6 large egg yolks, slowly adding 1 glass Madeira, 1 cup cold chicken broth, and 1 teaspoon ground cinnamon.

Smooth texture by passing through a sieve.

Cook gently in an earthen pot, stirring constantly, and adding a small pat of butter.

As it thickens, pour into cups and serve hot with a sprinkling of nutmeg and sugar.

Or try this:

Into a wine glass pour 1/4 glass Maraschino. Add 1 egg yolk (don't break it), add 1/4 glass mixed Madeira and Creme de Cacao. Then add 1/4 glass brandy.

Do not stir.
Drink in one gulp.

Why eggs?

An average egg will supply the body with 6.75 grams of the highest quality protein — its essential amino acids, the ones we cannot manufacture — all in the proper proportion for human tissue to utilize.

But . . . the eggs have to be fresh and free from the salmonella bacteria or you can get more than you bargain for!

Endive

German girls consider the endive to be a love charm.

Epimedium sagittatum

Barrenwort

This plant, common in China, was found to have aphrodisiac action when it was observed that goats feasting on it tended to copulate more frequently.

Eros

The Greek god of love.

Eruca sativa

Garden rocket

The ancient poets extolled the virtues of rocket for restoring vigor to sexual organs, tired of the tussle.

Dodens, 1586: "The use thereof stirreth up bodily pleasure, especially of the seed, also it provoketh urine, and helpeth the digestion of the meates".

Eryngo

Eryngium maritimum

Was Shakespeare versed in aphrodisiacs?

Falstaff implores, "Let the sky rain potatoes, let it thunder to the tune of Greensleeves, hail kissing comfits and stone eringoes: let there be a tempest of provocation . . . "

Comfits were holly roots which are candied to cover up the bitter, astringent taste. They were widely used in England to re-stimulate aged activity and encourage the young.

However, it was not every holly root that was so employed, it was the sea holly. The Greeks first discovered its ability to induce farts and the plant's name comes from the Greek "to eruct." Its use as a sexual stimulant was discovered later.

Try boiling two teaspoons of the little roots in a cup of water for five minutes or let them stand in wine for 1/2 an hour.

Essential Fatty Acids (EFA)

(See also Appendix, page 295)

Numerous clinical studies have assessed the cardioprotective effects of EFA's which have demonstrated the ability to reduce blood levels of LDL (low density lipoproteins) and increase the levels of HDL (high density lipoproteins). Although most of the research done has been concerned with heart disease, it has also been determined that HDL levels are statistically related to impotence.

Just as the heart needs unclogged blood vessels to receive an adequate supply of oxygen, so the penis requires open circulatory pathways to receive blood for an erection. And, just as fat in the bloodstream can build blockages in the arteries of the heart, so it can build blockages in the arteries supplying blood to the penis, interfering with the blood circulation. At that point, a kind of "heart attack" of the penis may occur, and a man may have difficilty having an erection.

An adequate amount of EFA's may lower the risk of impotency. Use two tablespoons daily of a high quality, cold-pressed vegetable oil, such as canola, or take two capsules of EPA fish oil capsules with each meal.

Eugenia crenulata

This herb's leaves steeped in rum form the basis of an aphrodisiac cocktail in Haiti.

Euphorbium

A gum resin derived from a plant found in South Africa. Avicenna mentions it as an aphrodisiac aid.

Exhalations

Body odors, both natural and perfumed, can produce marked impact on erotic manipulations.

Odors act powerfully upon the nervous system, they prepare it for all the pleasurable sensations, they communicate to it that slight disturbance or commotion which appears as if inseparable from emotions of delight, all which may be accounted for by their exercising a special action upon those organs, whence originated the most rapturous pleasure of which our nature is susceptible.

Foods for Love

Dr. Nicolas Venette, seventeenth century author of *Conjugal Love or The Pleasure of the Marriage Bed Reveal'd*, favors seminal strengtheners such as eggs, cock's testicles, crabs, prawns, beef marrow, crayfish, wine, milk and those foods which cause wind.

F

Fish and Venus

Fish have always been credited with aphrodisiac power. An explanation may be that Venus herself was born of the sea. More concrete explanations have to do with the nutritional value.

Flea-Wort

According to Pliny the Elder, the sap of this plant was an effective means of securing the birth of a boy. The aphrodisiac quality was a secondary value.

Fleeceflower Root

Polygonum multiflorum

The tubers of this plant are a favorite of Chinese herbalists.

Flowers

The aroma of certain flowers are aphrodisiacal. Particularly lilies of the valley, gardenia, henna, frangipani, and ylang-ylang.

Fly Agaric

Amanita muscaria

This mushroom is more of an hallucinogen than an aphrodisiac and an interesting ritual surrounding its use originated in the Koryak region of northeastern Siberia.

An early account of the orgiastic ritual states:

When they make a feast, they gather some of the mushrooms and boil them. They drink the water — chiefs and nobles get first crack — while the lower caste and low classes wait. As the orgy progresses, the desire to urinate overcomes the desire to copulate and the users pass water into special bowls. The active ingredient is still present in the urine so the lower castes can then also join in and partake.

This may be the plant from which Soma was derived in the Indus Valley of India. The chemistry indicates that it contains muscimol, a CNS hallucinogen, ibotenic acid, and muscayone. During the drying process other alkaloids are produced.

Fo-ti-tieng

According to Chinese herbalists, Li Ch'ung-yun, one of the originators of the Fo-ti-tieng formula, died at the advanced age of 256 years.

He imputed that part of his amazing lifespan and continued sexual vitality at his death (he had 24 wives), was due to a daily ration of Hydrocotyle asiatica minor. Scientists do not agree on the origin of the plant. Some say it is Gotu Kola (Centella asiatica) which is available at most herb and health stores in the U.S.

> *A daily cup of tea brewed from the leaves of Gotu Kola will boost sexual powers and contribute to resistance to disease and aging.*

Fo-ti-tieng is also available but whether it is the formula of Li or not is still a question.

Frangipane Cream

A pastry combining Frangipane, spices and almonds that is recommended as a sexual aid in an Italian erotic cookery manual.

Frankincense

This is the perfume also called olibanum that is frequently-mentioned in the Bible.

Fraxinus excelsior

European ash

The seeds, pickled in vinegar and salt, excite the appetite for food and love.

Frogs

The Romans used frogs and frog bones as sexual aids.

Fruits

Among fruits reputed to have stimulating qualities are bananas, figs, peaches, apples, cherries, grapes, and pomegranates.

Fugu

How far would you go for a night of amorous combat armed with a weapon that wouldn't flag but would stand erect for battle after battle?

Would you risk your life for such an experience?

Swimming in the sea off the coast of Japan is a tiny puffer fish, a blowfish with the capacity to invoke a major aphrodisiacal change in a man's nature.

This fish's flesh, when prepared correctly by a trained chef, is eaten raw as sashimi and its testicular fluid is blended with warmed saki and sipped.

Okay, so raw fish is not to everybody's taste but for a night of fantastic lovemaking, you'll get it down somehow.

But wait. There's a kicker!

Although certain parts of the fish will give you an erection that won't quit . . . other parts of the same fish contain a virulent poison. A quick-acting nerve toxin called tetradoxin. It is so virulent that it is said to be the main ingredient in the brew that makes a zombie of a human being. The merest trace of tetradoxin in the zombie formula destroys the will and leaves the user an automaton.

The preparation of the Fugu from sea to table requires the skill of a chef who has trained for years to earn a diploma in Fugu preparation. The edible portion and the poisonous are so intertwined that only the most highly trained eyes and the sharpest knife are able to separate a night of passion from the coldness of the grave.

If the chef has made an error, the diner will die in mid-mouthful . . . there is no known antidote.

Talk about coitus-interruptus . . . permanently!

Nevertheless, there are always people willing to bet their lives on the chance of that thrilling ultimate night of love. But before you book passage to Japan, you should be aware that about three hundred people so far got the last thrill of their lives because what should have been edible turned out to be tetradoxin!

Fumigation

Perfumed fumigation is used in Hindu erotology as a sexual stimulant.

G

Galanga

Kaempferia galanga
Maraba, China Root, India Root

Aleister Crowley used galanga in his formula for the *incense of Abremelin* in Liber AL III-23. This incense is used in Liber Samekh, a ritual designed for "Knowledge and Conversation" with your Holy Guardian Angel.

Maraba is used by natives in several parts of New Guinea for sexual fulfillment and as an hallucinogen.

The rhizome has been used in Ginger Beer in England and the chemistry of the volatile oils present in it has not been explored sufficiently, but galanga is a real, although relatively mild, hallucinogen.

A mixture of galanga, cubebs, sparrow wort, cardamoms, nutmeg, gillyflowers, Indian thistle, laurel seeds, cloves, and pepper is ground together and made into a tea. It is to be taken twice a day, morning and night, with chicken soup as an effective aphrodisiac.

Galega officinalis

Goat's rue

This herb has been offered by mail as the answer to a small bust. It has been sold with extreme discretion, via the mails, as a bust development miracle. Not only has it built many a bust but it is also claimed to be an aphrodisiac for the women who use it that way.

It has been used in Europe for centuries where it had been fed to cows to increase their milk yield by 30 to 50 percent.

Galium luteum

Lady's bedstraw

The roots of this herb, when beaten and macerated in wine, provoke lust.

Gall

The gall obtained from a jackal and rubbed into the penis made for a strong and compelling erection, according to Sheik Nefsawi, author of *The Perfumed Garden*.

Garcinia mannii

A small fruit tree found in West Tropical Africa. The fruit, similar to an orange but more acid in taste, is relished by the natives, while the roots — steeped in palm wine — are used as a sexual stimulant.

Garlic

Both European and Oriental erotologists consider garlic one of the best aphrodisiacs in the food category.

Gentian Wine

Considered to have the ability to inspire erections and amatory congress, particularly in an erotic atmosphere.

Gillyflower

This plant, long used as a condiment for its clove-scented leaves, is also used as a sexual stimulant when added to salads.

Ginger

Zingiber officianalis

In Senegal and French Guinea, ginger is chewed along with kola nut as a stimulant aphrodisiac.

The Chinese make a ginger jam that is used for the same reasons.

Arabs combine ginger with honey and pepper to make an amatory concoction.

Ginseng

Panax schinseng

One of the easiest herbs to obtain, since all herb stores and health food stores carry it in one form or another.

Ginseng is thought to be exclusively a Chinese herb but that isn't so. North American Indians used it before Europeans came to America. The Meskwaki Indians of Wisconsin combined ginseng, mica, gelatin and snake meat. It was prepared by the Indian women to "get a husband."

Or try this Chinese aphrodisiac mixture:

> *100 grams of ginseng, ginger, Atractylis ovata.*
> *Cook them in 8 quarts of water, boil down to 5 quarts.*
> *Drink 1 quart a day in three doses.*

Ginseng and its relative, Eleutherococcus senticosus, have been studied in Russia and in the U.S. for the past few years. Research has shown that it has body-building power. Also, that it is an adaptogen — a substance which helps the body adapt to stress.

Glycyrrhiza glabra

Licorice or sweet root

You are familiar with this herb since it is known all over the world because of its ability to soothe a sore throat or help calm a cough. The juice from licorice stains your teeth and tongue a temporary black and is one of the oldest known restoratives.

It's also a mild aphrodisiac!

Put 1/2 pound of dried root, chopped fine, into 3 quarts of water and boil down to 1 quart.

Strain, add milk and honey to taste.

In ancient Egypt, a herbal recipe for prolonged love goes this way:

Crush in a mortar:
1 ounce of fennel seed
1 ounce of sesame seed
1 ounce of licorice root
Then boil the mixture in a pint of water for five minutes.
Reduce heat — cover — simmer for twenty more minutes.
Let cool, strain and drink.

A recent analysis of licorice shows that it contains estrogenic substances.

Gossypion

A tree from which a juice is extracted. According to a medieval text by Andreas Cisalpinus, it was esteemed as an aphrodisiac.

Gourou

Resembles the horse chestnut. In the Sudan and Senegal, gourou is chewed for a type of general nervous stimulation which increases all of the physical abilities including the generative ones. It contains large amounts of caffeine and theobromine.

Grammatophyllum speciosum

Letter Plant

The natives of Malaysia and the Solomon Islands regard this fantastic orchid and the seeds it produces as the main ingredient for their love philtres.

Grape Juice

Squeezed directly from grapes into the mouth, it is said to be stimulating, particularly if unclad women are doing the squeezing.

Grewia umbellata

This herb is found in Siam, Sumatra and Borneo and used by the natives as a stimulant.

Grey

Lady Jane Grey was accused of bewitching King Edward VI by means of potions and amatory charms.

Guinea Fowl

French gourmets agree on guinea fowl roasted with truffles as a wonderful prelude to love.

Guarana

Like Maté, this is a caffeine-rich beverage from South America. It is made from the pulverized fruits of a vinelike plant that grows wild in the Amazon Valley and is also cultivated on small plantations. Guarana contains two to three times as much caffeine as coffee or tea. This makes it one of the most powerful of all caffeine drinks.

You don't have to go to the Amazon to get guarana. It's available in many health food stores, but go easy!

Havelock Ellis

With reference to cocoa, Havelock Ellis indicated that it was considered to come close to being an aphrodisiac beverage (as also chocolate). The Peruvian Indians described it as a stimulant tending to produce contractions of the womb, thereby increasing sexual activity.

King Henry VIII

King Henry VIII was no slouch in the bed chamber. His secret is not much of a secret since everyone can find it and use it at any time. It's parsley — the green leafy vegetable on your plate along with the hamburger that you carefully put to one side and then throw out.

H

Halibut

This fish, prepared with garlic and onions, is considered to have stimulating properties.

Haricot Beans

Like all beans, considered to be aphrodisiacal.

Harmine

Chemically related to mescaline and considered to be dangerous. It can be obtained from the plant *banisteria caapi* which grows in the foothills of the Andes and the Amazon basin. The leaves of the plant are plucked and then boiled in water to make a greenish infusion which contains the water soluble alkaloids. Harmine can also be derived from Wild Rue in Australia, New Zealand, and South America. It can produce strange hallucinations of a vivid, erotic nature.

Hashish

An Indian hemp plant, *cannabis indica*. In Arabic it means dried herb. It is chewed, smoked and drunk. The word assassin is derived from the Arabic hashishin, hemp eater.

Among Moroccans, a popular aphrodisiac is composed of a mixture of hashish, acorns, honey, sweet almonds, sesame, butter, nuts, and cantharides.

Hashish is able to remove both men and women's inhibitions and replace them with an uncontrollable excitement. It can be taken previous to a sexual liaison but is not really considered to be a true aphrodisiac. As inhibitions are removed, the user may incline towards sexual expression but no genital stimulation as such is involved.

Famous hashish addicts include Theophile Gautier, Balzac, Alexander Dumas, Baudelaire, and Charles Lamb.

Hedysarum

An old Oriental erotic text advises a mixture of the juices of Hedysarum gangeticum, the kuli and the kshirika plants in milk.

Heliotrope

Valeriana officinalis

A common garden plant that is a potent sedative and tranquilizer. Make a tea from the roots . . . but it stinks!

Hemp Pills

In Turkey, pills were composed of hemp buds, muscat nuts, ground fine and rolled in honey.

Henna

The powdered leaves and twigs of this plant are used as a hair dye. In early times it was thought that henna, rubbed on the fingers and the feet, stimulated lust.

Hibiscus cannabinus

The seeds can be eaten as sexual stimulants.

Hibiscus esculentus

Okra

In West Africa the seeds are considered to be stimulating.

In other parts of the world, okra, with its mucilaginous feel, is considered to be sexually stimulating. It is the main ingredient in gumbo soup.

Hindu Powder

An amatory powder can be made with the following:

Mix powdered Nelumbrium speciosum, blue lotus, and Mesna roxburghii and take with ghee and honey to excite the flesh.

Hippomanes

This is a protuberance that appears on a colt's head and is removed by the mare by biting it off soon after birth. The ancient Romans considered it to be a powerful sexual stimulant.

Honey

A compound of honey, ginger and pepper is recommended as an aphrodisiac by the thirteenth century Arab physician Avicenna.

Galen, a Greek of the second century A.D., physician to Emperor Marcus Aurelius, prepared an aphrodisiac for him of a glass of honey with almonds and pine nuts. It had to be taken for three days in a row.

Horseradish

This bitter herbal condiment is reputed to have a stimulating sexual effect.

Hygrophila spinosa

Seeds of this plant mixed with sugar, milk and wine, have been used to combat impotence.

I

Iboga

Tabernanthe iboga

The root bark of an equatorial African herb is used in Gabon as an aphrodisiac. It increases temperature, blood pressure and glandular activity. Its use is said to kindle a passion that persists for the better part of a day, even after only taking one gram of the root. Fortunately or unfortunately, the U.S. has placed it on the Drug Enforcement Agency's list of controlled substances. Therefore, you'll have to pick it up in Mexico, or on one of your other holiday trips and leave yourself adequate time to enjoy its effects.

Imperatoria ostruthium

Masterwort

A decoction of the root in wine can revive an almost extinct inclination and ability to copulate.

Intestines

The intestines of fish and birds were used as aphrodisiacs among the Romans.

Ipomoea digitata

Fingerleaf morning glory

Powder the root and macerate it in the juice of the stem, then mix it with ghee and honey for use as an aphrodisiac.

Italian aphrodisiac soup

The recipe involved calf's heel, crayfish, carrots, celery and shallots.

J

Jasminum grandiflorum

Arab books mention the use of this flower applied as a plaster to the loins, genitals, and pubes as an aphrodisiac.

Jimson Weed

Thorn Apple, Devil's Trumpet, Yerba del Diablo

With its large, thin, dark-green leaves and bell-shaped white or light purple flowers, this rank-smelling plant is easily identified as *Datura stramonium*. A member of the potato family, relative of belladonna, mandrake, and henbane, and loaded with alkaloids such as atropine, hyoscyamine, mandragorine and scopalamine.

A bummer of a hallucinogenic trip can be the result of a large dose. Tiny, tiny doses may be useful but not worth the potential danger.

Jugulans regia

Walnuts are high in nutritional value, including the sex mineral phosphorus, and have a reputation for having aphrodisiac properties.

Juniper

This shrub produces purple berries of a fleshy consistency with a pungent taste. The oil is used in medicine, in cordials, and in love philtres as a means of maintaining youthful ardor.

Juno virginesis

The Romans called her the goddess who ruled over the consummation of marriage.

Louis XIV, The Sun King (1638-1715)

Although facially scarred by a childhood bout with smallpox, Louis was a charmer and an indefatigable lover. Married twice, he had innumerable affairs and was an equal opportunity lover. Palace servants and noblewomen graced his bed. His sexual appetite was fueled by copious amounts of meat and fowl usually cooked in wine and spiced to the taste of the king.

K

Kama

A Sanskrit term used to express sexual pleasure.

Kama Sutra

A Sanskrit manual of erotic procedures, written by Vatsyayana and translated into English by Sir Richard Burton.

Kantaka

In the Kama Sutra, a means of increasing vigor is this mixture:

Powder of milk hedge plant
Powder of kantaka plant
Powder of lanjalika plant
Monkey excrement
Mix together and take three nights in a row.

Kava Kava

Piper methysticum (See also *"Kava Kava", page 39)*

Previously written about but here's a footnote. Before the missionaries came to the South Pacific, Kava Kava enjoyed the widest popularity. The missionaries convinced the natives that the pleasure-giving drink should be forbidden. So it was, and the natives replaced it with alcohol which is far more dangerous and more likely to be addictive. Nowadays, Kava Kava is making a well-received comeback and is actually being used to wean alcoholics away from the Western-inspired habit of alcoholism.

Khat

Catha edulis

To Yemenites and some East Africans, khat is the answer nature has provided to the use of amphetamines. Khat can keep you awake and alert until dawn and make you explosively sexier every minute of those hours. It is also a weight-loss marvel — absolutely no willpower necessary. Natives chew the young buds, fresh leaves and stems of the plant, or brew them into a tea which is imbibed on a regular basis similar to the coffee drinkers of the Western world. But . . . that's where the similarity ends. Khat is more dangerous than coffee. It can be all of the good things, but it can also be a bad trip and it is much more habit-forming than coffee. Maybe that's the reason it's no longer available in the U.S.

Kidneys

The kidneys of sheep, pigs and cattle are believed to be able to increase the sexual function.

Kitab Al-lzah Fi'ilm Al-Nikah

An Arabic manual on sex written by Jalai al-Din al-Siyuti.

Kite

In Hindu erotic literature, a mixture of honey and the prickly hairs of the cowach — a tropical pod — plus the remains of a dead kite help sexual union.

Kosth

In the *Anaga-Ranga* there is a formula for increasing the strength of the male member with kosth. This is the way it is made:

> *Mix costus arabicus, lechi, chikana, askhand, kanher root, gajapimpali together in butter and apply to the genitals.*

Most of the ingredients are indigenous to India.

Kuili

A means of recovering sexual vigor in older males is offered in the *Ananga-Ranga* as follows:

> *Kuili powder, Kanta-gokhru, lechi, Asparagus racemosus, and cucumber mixed in milk and taken daily at bedtime.*

Most of the ingredients are from India.

Kuttanimatam

A Hindu manual on sexual techniques by Dhamodaragupta. It has been translated into English and French.

And Yet Women Still Complain

Apuleius — second century A.D. — was reputed to have used cuttlefish, spiced oysters, hedgehogs, and lobsters to gain the love of a widow.

From Shakespeare's Troilus and Cressida

Cressida:

All lovers swear more performance than they are able,
And yet reserve an ability that they never perform,
Vowing more than the performance of ten,
And discharging less than the tenth part of one.

L

Lamprey

An eel-like sucker fish frequently found in the company of sharks. A soup which includes this sea creature is said to increase the production of seminal fluid.

Lard

This animal fat mixed with chopped garlic has been used as an erotic ointment to increase slippery union and prolonged erections.

Laurel leaves

Oriental books extol laurel tea as a sexual stimulant.

Lavender

Besides the pleasant smell, a mixture of lavender and tobacco, when smoked, excites the senses.

Lee

William H. Lee, Ph.D., pharmacist, nutritionist, medical herbalist of the twentieth century. With his wife and partner, Lynn, they wrote *Herbal Aphrodisiacs, New Power To Love,* and this book, *The Encyclopedia of Concentrated Aphrodisiacs.*

Lentils

This food was believed to stimulate desire by the ancient Greeks.

Leonorus sibiricus

Siberian motherwort

The seeds are chewed for a loss of virility, to prevent contraceptions.

Lepidium sativum

Garden cress

A preparation made of the seeds, sugar and clarified butter is used in India to treat general debility.

For flagging sexual energy, try mixing the pulverized seeds, coconut, jaggery, sugar and milk. For extra strength add some licorice root.

Licorice

Glycyrrhiza glabra
Sweet Root

Previously discussed, but the Scythians could live on cheese and licorice tea on fortnight marches, and in India, licorice milk and honey was a favorite pre-amour cocktail.

Liébault, Jean

French sexologist and author of *Thresor des Remedes Secrets pour Les Maladies des Femmes,* translated into French from his original works in Latin in 1582.

It is an encyclopedia of sexual knowledge as it was known in his time. Detailed suggestions were written on how to strengthen sexual vigor, and here is a sound and wholesome diet with recipes to reinforce erotic feelings.

Nuts, dates, figs, wine in moderation, fish cooked in onions, pomegranates, chestnuts, chicken soup, spices and rice cooked in milk were part of his suggestions.

Lingam Preparation

Applications to the penis prior to love included these from the *Ananga-Ranga*:

> *Honey, goose fat, butter, storax, ghee, spurge chives, musk, ginger, ambergris, pepper, anise, rui seed, lotus flower pollen.*

Lion's Fat

Lion's fat was a popular aphrodisiac in medieval times.

Liver

Calf's liver, according to Horace, was popular in his day as an aphrodisiac.

Lizard

Any lizard will do for this recipe:

> *Pound together a lizard, cubebs, ginger, cardamom, pepper, cloves, cinammon, opium and boil the entire mass in olive oil. Then add frankincense and coriander. Macerate the dish in heavy honey.*

On the night before amour, eat the entire lizard, washed down with wine and followed with rose sherbet.

Lobelia inflata

Indian tobacco

Although this herb has been smoked to get a marijuana-like high, it can also be turned into a drink.

> *One tablespoon of crushed leaves to a pint of water. Simmer, strain and take a drink.*

Lonicera japonica

Honeysuckle

The use of flowers, leaves and vine are said to be prolonging agents to vitality. The flowers and leaves have long been used in the Orient to make a pleasant tasting tea.

Lozenges

Pastilles, perfumed with ambergris, were sold as aphrodisiac aids.

Lycium chinense

Chinese tea-tree

Chinese herb which is said to have a considerable effect upon the genitourinary system. One of the prized Oriental herbs that is available at most herb shops and health food stores.

Lady Jane Grey

The unfortunate Lady was accused of bewitching King Edward VI of England by preparing amatory meals. Because of this she was beheaded. All she prepared was tasty dinners with Indian spices.

Lycopodium

Plant with a claw-like root used in pharmacies in the early part of this century to keep suppositories from sticking to each other when placed in a box. It was thought of as an aphrodisiac in ancient times.

M

Madhuca latifolia

Butter tree

Mix the flowers with milk to help with impotence caused by a general debility.

Mammea americana

Mamey

A fruit tree native to the West Indies. The fruit was considered to be so potent and stimulating that only men were permitted to eat it. They sliced it and served it with sugar, cream and wine as a preparation for sex.

Mango

Some Hindus use the mango in the following manner:

> *Arris root is dressed with mango and placed in the hole in the trunk of the Sisu tree for six months. Then, when retrieved, it is made into an ointment and applied to the genitalia for a sustained erection.*

Manichaeans

St. Augustine accused this religious sect of practicing rites associated with erotic perversions.

Maté

Millions of people in South America enjoy a cup of maté in the same manner as coffee or tea. The aromatic flavor and the uplifting caffeine can be easily extracted from the dried leaves by pouring water, hot or cold, over a small pile of them.

The youngest leaves offer the best quality, while the cheaper grades contain twigs, stems and older leaves. Botanically, maté is a species of holly.

Marjoram

This spice is said to have aphrodisiac value.

Marrow

Bone marrow is a source of vitality according to many old traditions. A paté of bone marrow was considered elemental for whetting the amorous appetite.

Marzipan

In *Gargantua and Pantagruel,* Rabelais recommends a slice of marzipan and a drink of hippocras (red Burgundy wine, plus ginger, crushed cinnamon, cloves, vanilla and sugar), as amatory ammunition.

Masochism

Sexual pleasure derived from the infliction of pain or cruelty upon oneself. Originated in the name of the Austrian novelist Leopold von Sacher-Masoch.

Mastic

A drink made from the fruit of the mastic tree, mixed with honey and olive oil, was used by the Arabs as a means of increasing sperm production.

Matico

Piper angustifolium

This pepper shrub grows to a height of eight feet in its native Peru. The Indians regard it as an effective aphrodisiac and use it in the following manner:

> *Take a tablespoon of the dried leaves and boil for one minute. Then, let steep for about a half-hour. Strain. Add honey to taste and drink cold.*

Matricaria chamomilla

German chamomile

Although it is usually associated with a calming action to the nerves and the digestive tract, when applied as a strong tea to the genitals it is said to have a stimulating effect.

Meat

Lean red meat is credited with having a strong aphrodisiac effect.

Medea

Ancient witch found in Greek and Roman mythology. One of her specialties was the restoration of virility by means of charms and potions. The Greek poet, Euripides, in his tragic drama *Medea,* has her encouraging the aged Aegeus.

"Thus by the gods shall thy desire of children be accomplished to thee, and thou thyself shalt die in happiness. But thou knowest not what this fortune is that thou hast found; but I will free thee from being childless, and I will cause thee to raise up offspring — such charms I know."

Membrum

The hedgehog and the wolf were not very lucky in ancient Rome since their genital organs were among the ingredients specified in many Roman philtres.

Mens Sana

Juvenal, the Roman writer, realized that the opinion that a good physical and psychological condition was necessary for sexual joy was correct and coined the phrase, "*Mens sana in corpore sano.*" A healthy mind in a healthy body.

Why Eat Meat?

It's true that many authorities advise against eating meat to excess.

However, if you trim the visible fat, prepare it correctly, avoid the use of too much salt, and avoid eating it every day, meat will contribute valiantly to your sex life.

How?

Let's talk brain chemistry again.

Protein is composed of amino acids.

Amino acids are the body's building block and tissue restoratives. They repair worn tissue, make new cells, and manufacture chemical messengers.

While your body can make some of the amino acids from foods, it cannot manufacture the "essential amino acids." Those must be obtained from the food you eat.

Meat contains the amino acids phenylalanine and tyrosine. The brain uses these amino acids to make the stimulating chemical messenger called norepinephrine. Norepinephrine influences the baser, sexier impulses. It makes a person more aggressive, more willing to take risks, more of a fighter and a lover.

Mentha species

Mint of all types

All mints are useful as stomachics but there are those people who react to the vibrant taste and stimulating aroma with a longing for love.

Meum athamanticum

Bawdwort

The root, boiled in water as a tea, stimulates the genitourinary tract.

Miletus

An ancient, wealthy city of Ionia in Asia Minor known for the preparation of aphrodisiac apparatus.

Milk

Arab tradition has it that bathing the genitals with asses' milk stimulated vigor. Nero's wife bathed in asses' milk because Poppaea thought it increased her sensuality and beauty.

Minerals

(See also Appendix, page 297)

Vitamins get the publicity but minerals make the difference.

Calcium — essential to the healthy functioning of muscles, nerves, heart, stamina, energy. Helps to control or release passion. Balances glands.

Chromium — helps regulate blood sugar, therefore the amount of sexual energy available.

Germanium — is said to affect sexual impulses.

Iodine — an underactive thyroid gland can result in the loss of the sex drive altogether. Thyroid must have iodine.

Iron — a lack of iron is accompanied by fatigue and a loss of interest in sexual activity.

Phosphorus — essential to sexual activity. Without phosphorus, no sex life is possible. As much as 80% of the male sex fluid is lecithin which contains a great deal of phosphorus.

Potassium — affects sexuality by insuring healthy nerve and muscle activity. Without sufficient potassium you would be too weak and uncoordinated to have sex at all.

Silicon — an enjoyable sex life is impossible without an abundance of silicon. The outer sheaths of the nerves need silicon to be active.

Sodium — all body fluids need sodium including the sexual fluids. Sex is impossible without it.

Sulfur — helps keep the sexual parts of the body free of impurities.

Zinc — is needed by the prostate gland, sperm cells, and plays an important role in the maintenance of the sexual system.

Mixoscopy

Voyeurism. Secret observation of the sexual act designed to stimulate the observer in an erotic manner.

In legend, according to Homer's *Odyssey,* Hephaestus, husband to Aphrodite, invited the gods to observe her conduct as she made love to Aries, the god of war.

Moh

Bassia latifolia

This tree grows flowers that are rich in natural sugar. In India, these flowers are fermented to make a liquor named *arrack*.

The *Ananga-Ranga* recommends the pith of this tree be pounded with cow's milk as a remedy for the loss of virility.

Mollusca

The mollusca and testaceous animals are useful in restoring potency.

Momordica balsamina

Balsam pear

The root of this vine has been used as an ingredient in a number of aphrodisiacal recipes.

Mormon Tea

Ephedra nevadensis

Chinese ephedra has been used for more than 5,000 years. In 2700 B.C., Shen Mung, the father of Chinese medicine, used the dried roots and stems as a decongestant to treat coughs and colds. However, it is as a fermented drink that is used as a stimulant for other purposes.

The Chinese technique is to put an ounce of the herb into boiling water, let boil covered for five minutes, then turn off the heat and let stand. Cool, strain, add honey to taste. This tea should not be used if one suffers from high blood pressure, diabetes, heart disease or has problems with the thyroid. In fact, none of these preparations should be used if there is any medical involvement unless your doctor agrees.

Mucun pruriens

Cowhage

The hairs of the pod are used to get rid of worms in the stomach in India but the seeds, powdered and mixed with honey, are used as a aphrodisiac.

Mugwort

This plant was associated with amatory tendencies in some areas of the Orient.

Muira Puama

This is the scraped-out inner bark of the tree known as *Lyriosma ovata*. The native Jivaro Indians chew on the fresh plant as a stimulant aphrodisiac but the dried bark is in the Brazilian pharmacopoeia as a remedy for impotence.

Externally, it is used as a strong decoction and rubbed on the genitals. Internally, it is used as a fluid extract with doses of about fifteen drops daily.

In the sixties, a firm in Germany advertised a mixture of this herb with testicular tissue, anterior pituitary extract, lecithin, cola extract, yohimbine, calcium lactate, and strychnine. It was touted as a rejuvenation product.

The active ingredient, while somewhat soluble in water is very soluble in alcohol. An alcoholic solution of the powdered herb is apt to be too strong for most users and can cause stomach upset or anti-social behavior.

> *Steep a half-ounce of the herb in vodka for a week, then strain after shaking. Take a shot or two daily but don't overdo.*

Mushrooms

Arabs considered the eating of mushrooms an aid to lovemaking.

Musk

Genuine musk is derived from the glands of the male musk deer found in the Himalayas. When taken internally, it is as aphrodisiac in power as ambergris. Externally, it produces mountainous erections of singular ability. It is said to have restored the powers of his youth to an eighty-year-old man. It is also said to be as useful when obtained from a species of goat native to the Tartars.

The odor of musk, according to the *Kama Sutra,* is associated with the ideal woman.

Musk Seed

Abelmoschus or Hibiscus moschatus

There is an evergreen shrub native to Asia but now grown and cultivated in India, Egypt and the West Indies, that has seeds the size of large lentils. These seeds smell like musk, have a sweet taste and mix well with coffee, chocolate, or as a delightful tea alone.

They have an intoxicating sex-stimulating aroma which contributes to their aphrodisiacal power. Grind the seeds and make an emulsion with milk or try to get the concentrated tincture in an Indian shop.

Mustard

Hot mustard baths were recommended for women who had difficulty in responding to men.

Mustela Piscis

The brains were considered to be a sexual stimulant to women. Prepared as a broth or mixed with garlic and onions, they were used as an excitant.

Mutton

Among certain Arab tribes, mutton mixed well with ground caraway seed was a potent beginning to a night of romance.

Myrrh

Eggs, boiled with myrrh, pepper and cinnamon, eaten on seven successive days, assured the eater of fantastic feats of extended love.

Myrtle

In the Middle Ages, people used the pulverized leaves as an application to the body. This acted as a sexual stimulant.

A love tonic was made from myrtle as follows:

> *Use the flowers and leaves, two handfuls, infuse them in two quarts of spring water and one quart of white wine for 24 hours. Strain. Mix the myrtle water with a good cordial and drink.*

This will make those who imbibe very amorous.

Myrtus communis

Myrtle leaves mixed with delicate cordials are said to incline the drinker to amorous thought and coital conditions.

George IV

This English king so highly appreciated the ability of mushrooms, particularly truffles, to prepare him for sexual combat that his ministers at the Court of Turin, Naples and Florence were instructed to forward to the Royal Kitchen any truffles found that were superior in flavor and delicacy.

N

Nandina domestica

Evergreen shrub with shiny, red berries found in hilly areas in China. The seeds have the ability to strengthen virility.

Nasturtium officinale

Watercress

The seeds have been found to be stimulant in nature.

Necks of Fattened Snails

Ancient Romans considered snail necks soaked in wine to be an aphrodisiac.

Nedde

A mixture of various perfumes plus benzoin and amber is used to anoint various points in the body to excite lust as the partner attempts to locate all odorous portions with his tongue.

Nefzawi

Umar ibn Muhammed al-Nefzawi, the author of *The Perfumed Garden,* lived in Tunisia. The book ranges in contents from sexual physiology to copulation. Medicines, aphrodisiacs, and sexual rites are discussed in great detail.

Nelumbium nucifera

Chinese lotus

The marble-sized seeds can be eaten raw, candied, roasted, or boiled for their libido-enriching power.

Nepenthes

A drug mentioned by Homer in *The Odyssey* as having the effect of banishing sorrow or mental trouble. It has been identified witha number of materials, principally opium, hashish, or *Panax chironium.*

Theophrastus, Greek philosopher, third century B.C., suggested that it was an aphrodisiac when mixed with wine.

Newbouldia laevis

Africans use the roots and leaves for their aphrodisiacal ability.

Night-Blooming Cereus

Selenicereus grandiflorus

This is a fleshy cactus with flowers that grow to a foot or more in size and smell like vanilla when they first open their leaves to the moon. Soon after, they dry up. Six hours of life and then they are gone. But, they leave their stems and the stems are what herbalists are after. The stems and sometimes the flowers are useful in cases of sexual inability due to exhaustion.

A half-gram of fresh stem may be chewed, or 5 drops of the fresh juice will do the trick.

Too much, however, will cause stomach upset and put all thoughts of sex out of your mind. Start with the lowest dosage until you can gauge its effect.

Ninjin

This root, highly regarded in Japan as an aphrodisiac, is not identified completely. Some say it is the Mandrake root since the properties are somewhat similar.

Nuoc-Man

An aphrodisiac sauce consisting of decayed fish as a base. The aphrodisiac elements are phosphorus and salt, naturally present in the fish, and the other added ingredients. It is much in use in the Far East, especially among the Chinese. In Vietnam, the sauce is seasoned with pimento and garlic. Many servicemen have come across it while on a tour of duty but it has not found favor with Americans because of its flavor.

Nutmeg

An aromatic seed of a tree that is native to the East Indies. It is used to spice food and is one of the popular ingredients in egg nog. It is highly prized in the Orient as an aphrodisiac. Too much can be dangerous.

Nutrition

Experiments have shown that sexual interest and desire increase with nutritional satisfaction, and that, inversely, a lowering of nutritional values coincides with a diminution of sex expression. As a rule, therefore, any kind of faulty nutrition will affect sexual ability.

For continued virility, a balanced diet plus the proper supplemental vitamins and minerals are of utmost importance.

Certain foods and food combinations, besides providing balanced nutrition, help to increase sexual desire and ability by overloading the body with those elements designed to act as stimulants.

Menus designed with erotology in mind can be the basis of a hearty diet and also be stimulating.

Nux vomica

Contains strychnine. Use of this plant can increase muscle tone and rigidity; therefore, this poison can act as an aid to an increase in erectile tissue. The trouble is, you can die with an erection!

This is dangerous and should be left alone.

Nymphaea

This is an aphrodisiac in the form of an ointment which is applied to the body. It is composed of oil of hogweed, echites putescens, the sarina plant, yellow amaranth, and nymphaea leaves ground together and mixed with lard.

Nymphs

In Greek mythology, the nymphs roamed the forests and streams in search of handsome youths to favor with their love. Sometimes the satyrs of the woods won their favor. They were the symbols of sexual provocation and sexual pleasure.

Catherine the Great

Certainly, Catherine the Great will go down in history for many adventures, including her dalliance with a mule which cost her dearly, but when she was desperate to bring an heir into this world, she turned to the ocean. Her husband having failed his marital duty, she turned to one of her royal guards (Saltokoff by name), some caviar, a large helping of sturgeon, and soon became "Mother Russia."

O

Octopus

The octopus, and sometimes just the sepia ink, was considered to be an aphrodisiac by the ancient Romans. Try it with cooked onions, oil, pepper and vinegar.

Oilbanum

This is an aromatic resin once valued as a medicine. It is used today as an incense but the Greeks and Romans considered it to be an aphrodisiac.

In the Bible, oilbanum was called frankincense and was prized for its pleasant and stimulating odor. Among the Turks, an exciting compound of oilbanum, myrrh, camphor, and musk was made to cause a strong stimulation to the genitals.

Old Oriental Recipe

> *Tuccinum bole, musk, ambergris, aloe, red and yellow saunders, mastic, sweetflag, galanga, cinnamon, rhubarb, myrobalon, absinthe, pounded on precious stones.*

This prescription imparts a sweetness to the breath and an urgency to the loins.

Olouiqui

Rivea corymbosa

This is the Aztec mind-altering seed. It is native to the mountains of Mexico, a member of the bindweed family, and a more or less pleasant intoxicant. The active ingredient is d-lysergic acid, just a bit milder than lysergic acid.

Soak about ten crushed seeds in water and have a drink. For the next six hours, after some stomach upset, you should enjoy sex, tripping, hallucinations and a good night's sleep.

If you have ever had any problems with your liver this is not for you. First trippers should bring along a guide.

Onions

The onion and other bulbous, smelly plants have a reputation for possessing aphrodisiac qualities. The poet Ovid, in his *Remedy for Love,* recommends onions and garlic. Martial, the Roman epigrammatist, advises, if your wife is old and your member exhausted, eat onions in plenty.

A later poet, Columella, declared that onions inflame and animate girls.

For men, onions add virility, for women they purify the blood.

Onions and egg yolks are a dish prepared by the Arabs to stimulate virility, and Oriental dishes intended to be aphrodisiacs frequently contain onions.

Onion Seed

In the famous book on love, *The Perfumed Garden,* Nefzawi proposes this sexual stimulant:

> *Pound onion seeds until they are powdered.*
> *Sift to remove the outer shell*
> *Mix well with honey and take only this for 24 hours.*

Another recommended dish for sexual potency is onions boiled with condiments and aromatic spices, then fried in olive oil and the yolks of eggs. This preparation is to be taken on several successive days for best results, although even one dish will be the beginning of a sustained erection.

According to the Greek physician Galen, the onions should first be pounded to make them easier to digest and then eaten with unclarified honey.

Opium

Papaverum somniferum

Opium gets its start as the milky juice from the unripe capsule of the poppy. After the petals fall off, slits are made in the pods to let the sap drip out. The sap is collected and dried in the sun to make a black tar-like substance.

This substance contains codeine, morphine and papaverine. Papaverine is not a narcotic but a muscle relaxant.

Opium was known to the ancient Sumerians who called it "plant of joy." Primarily, opium has been known for its ability to relieve pain and cause sleep with dreams. However, in small doses there is a stimulation of the spinal nerves that control blood flow and erection of both the penis and the clitoris. So, while the rest of your body, and her body, is becoming more and more relaxed, both of your essential sexual areas are becoming more and more aroused. Along with that is another phenomena. By using a small amount of opium, the surface nerves of the penis and the clitoris are less sensitive although the deeper layers are more active. This gives you, the owners of these areas, a far greater control over the time of release than you have ever had in the past.

Thus, you can choose to delay climax as long as you want, right up to the moment that mutual sexual tension is almost unbearable.

This is not a drug to be abused, since frequent use will result in the opposite effect until there is no desire for sex at all.

The best way to use opium for sexual pleasure is with a suppository. In that way, the nausea associated with it can be avoided. If it is eaten, the body converts some of the morphine to apomorphine which is a strong emetic. The anal route avoids the hydrochloric acid in the stomach which is the converting factor. Also, the results can begin in as little as fifteen minutes because you apply it right next to the area that is pumped up by its powers. The amount needed is less than the size of a pea but, in sensitive individuals, even that can still cause trouble.

Sexual disinterest and even genital atrophy can be side effects of overuse. Even a couple of days indulgence will attack the immune system and lower your resistance to colds and infections and it is illegal!

Tantric yoga will take you along the same path without the side effects and without fear of the law.

Opium smoking, while generally thought of in connection with China, was not introduced into China until Emperor Ch'ung Ch'en outlawed tobacco in the seventeenth century. It did not become big business there until the British forced the trade on China in the Opium War.

Dioscorides described its attributes in the first century A.D.

Thomas De Quincey, the English essayist, was an opium user for some twenty-five years. It was first prescribed to ease the pain of a toothache.

The Hindu name for opium is chandu and it is both eaten and smoked for vitality.

Homer, in *The Iliad* writes:

> *Down sank his head, as in a garden sinks*
> *a ripened poppy charged with venal rains;*
> *So sank his head beneath his helmet's weight.*

Hippocrates, the Greek physician, recommended poppy juice in the fifth century.

Pliny the Elder considered the poppy to be a valuable medicine.

Vespucci mentions opium as part of a cargo brought from India to Lisbon in 1501.

In Biblical times, King David, who was subject to fits of depression, took a potion which consisted in part of opium.

In Ancient Egypt, poppy seeds were mixed with flour and honey as a wedding cake.

The Emperor Nero used potions compounded with poppy.

Theophrastus refers to the use of opium as a medicine against pain and depression.

Laudanum, a derivative of opium, was the name given to an opium compound by Paracelsus in the sixteenth century.

Opotherapy

The use of extracts and juices of the genital glands of animals to re-stimulate sexual activity in those whose natural ability has been lost through time or overuse.

The extracts contain the sexual hormones of the animals and may be of value to stimulate sexual congress.

Orchid

These plants have anatomical similarity to genitalia and in Greek the name means *testes*. Therefore, in fact and in legend, the orchid has been used as a sexual stimulant.

Orchis hircina

In ancient times the root of this plant was the basis of a powerful aphrodisiac called Satyrion.

Orchis Morio

A plant of the satyrion species, used in Turkey as a stimulant. Its natural habitat is the mountains in the vicinity of Istanbul.

Organotherapy

In sexual disorders, the treatment consists, in one direction, of the consumption of the genitalia of animals — stags, roosters, asses — as a means of recovering sexual potency.

The testes of animals were also used for this purpose, and meals were compounded mainly of these ingredients. The practice was common in India and the Orient as well as among the ancient Romans.

Origanum majorana

Marjoram

This plant shows a distinct relationship to the sexual organs. Sexual excitement, particularly among women, results from the use of this herb. Lascivious dreams and increased desire for coitus is the usual result.

Orobanche ammophyla

This plant was thought to spring up from the semen of wild stallions. The plant or the root are eaten raw or cooked with partridge or other fowl. It is considered to be one of the better aphrodisiacs.

P

Padmini

The Lotus-Woman. In Hindu erotic literature, she is the ideal woman. She has all of the emotional and physical characteristics of feminine seductiveness.

Pan

Greek god of the forest, mountain and streams whose dominant characteristic is a continual desire for lovemaking. He has the feet of a goat, an indication of vast amorous propensity.

His flock includes satyrs who are equally interested in lustful pursuits. Pan, in Greek, means everything, and the implication is that the entire world . . . the entire cosmos is permeated and conditioned by the procreative force.

Panax quinquefolia

American ginseng

China is the best customer for American and Canadian ginseng which they say is almost as good as their homegrown variety. It has all of the qualities of the Chinese variety and is as effective as a sexual stimulant.

Pandanus odoratissimus

Screwpine

The younger flower spikes are pounded and boiled with milk in Malaysia as a love potion.

Pannychis

A Greek festival honoring Aphrodite, goddess of love. During this festival, prostitutes, and other ladies, roamed the darkened streets offering their favor for a small sum so that all could join in the celebration.

Paprika

A red pepper grown in Hungary and imbued with the ability to arouse lust.

Paracelsus

Occultist of the sixteenth century who wrote about and prepared amatory potions, among other pursuits.

Partes Genitales

These organs, particularly of the cock, can be powerful aphrodisiacs according to Mery, in the book *Traité Universel des Drogues Simples*.

Parthenius

Native of Nicaea who lived and wrote in the first century B.C. Noted for a collection of love stories which became an amatory reference work.

Pastinaca sativa

Parsnip

While the root may be eaten and it is very nourishing, it is the seed which is used as an aphrodisiac. It is powdered and heated in water, then filtered and taken to arouse a tired member.

Pastry

The Chinese and the Arabs considered food to serve a double purpose, nourishment and sexual stimulation. In that light, pastries were commonly used as aphrodisiacs.

Honey, ginger, vinegar, pellitory, cardamom, garlic, cinnamon, pepper, nutmeg, hellebore were mixed together into a cake as a specific cure for impotency.

In the Middle Ages, the practice of mixing particular aphrodisiacs into bread and pastries intended for the stimulation of a person was widely used at intimate suppers. The person would respond to the amorous attention of the party-giver without knowing that he or she had been force-fed stimulating spices or other sexually provocative material.

Pauravisia

In Melanesian mythology, the phallic snake.

Peas

Peas may be food to you but to Nefzawi, of *The Perfumed Garden*, the preparation determines the outcome.

To create passion, prepare your peas this way:

> *Fresh, young green peas boiled with onions, powdered with cinnamon, ginger and cardamom will revive even the most tired of penile members.*

Peaches

Of stimulating aphrodisiac value when ripe and full of nutritive elements.

Pellitory

Anacyclus pyrethrum

It looks a lot like chamomile but it was used as a love stimulant not a digestant by the ancient Romans. As a means of raising the lance again, Ovid writes of pellitory root steeped in wine.

Penianthus patulinervis

The roots or the young twigs are made into a decoction by the people of Sierra Leone as an aphrodisiac.

Pepper

In general, pepper is useful as a condiment. Combined with nettle-seed it has exciting sexual properties. White or red pepper has been written about although black pepper may have the same effect.

Perch

In the head of this fish are said to be small stone-like objects which are used to concoct love philtres.

Perfumed Bed

In the Bible, mention is made of the use of perfume in connection with the adulterous woman.

> *I have perfumed my bed with myrrh, aloes, and cinnamon.*
> *Come, let us take our fill of love until the morning:*
> *Let us solace ourselves with loves.*
>
> Proverbs: 7; 17-18

Perfumed Genitalia

From the earliest times in Egypt, Alexandria, France . . . women have made a practice of using perfumed pads. Their intention was to arouse the utmost sensory excitation in their lovers. The perfumed sacs were used in the *pudenda muliebria*.

Perfumes

Among the ancient Romans, in particular, erotic impulses were encouraged by the use of scent. Perfumes were applied to the body, the head, to garments and to bedsheets. Civet and ambergris were popular among the wealthy. Aromatic spices perfumed the breath. Myrrh, cinnamon, sweet marjoram were to be found everywhere.

Arab erotic books speak of the importance of perfumes for men and women as an indirect and subtle stimulant in amorous techniques.

Ruth anointed herself with fragrant oils.

Esther purified herself with myrrh and sweet odors.

Judith anointed herself with precious ointments.

Alexander the Great perfumed himself with violets.

Persea americana

Avocado

The pulp of the avocado is credited with having the ability to stimulate sexual congress. Avocados are a good source of phosphorus, sulphur, magnesium and other important minerals.

Persian Formula

Take cloves, cinnamon and cardamom and put them in a jar. Fill the jar with rosewater and steep your husband's shirt in it with a piece of parchment inscribed with his name. Heat everything over a fire, and as it boils so will his love increase to boiling.

Perspiration

Often has a powerful impact. Henry III of Navarre inadvertently inspired a passion in Maria of Cleves and Henry IV in Gabrielle through the transmission of a handkerchief used to wipe away perspiration.

Or so they say!

Petroselinum hortense

Parsley

The seed of the parsley, ground in wine, increases the sexual appetite of women.

Petits Parfums

Ingenious way in which sixteenth century professional beauties in France retained or acquired the love of a selected man. They filled tiny bags with musk and by bursting these bags at appropriate moments, the women enveloped their lovers in a provocative, sexually arousing atmosphere.

Pheasant

The roasted flesh of the pheasant was considered to be highly aphrodisiac in effect.

Most game is traditionally associated with amatory effects.

Philodemus

Philodemus of Gadara was a Greek Epicurean philosopher of the first century B.C. He wrote a collection of erotic poetry which ranged over the entire field of sexual exercise and variety including orgiastic and drunken revels, perversions, and every type of lewdness.

Philostratus

Greek writer of ancient times, author of *The Life of Apollonius of Tyana*, full of erotic stories and all sorts of amatory situations.

Philtre

Any magic potion intended to have an amorous effect on the drinker. The ancient Romans and Greeks knew a great deal about the aphrodisiac purposes of such potions. Plutarch mentions them in *Marriage Precepts*.

The ingredients could be exotic or repulsive depending on the formula. They could be bones of frogs or sparrows, betel nuts, genitals, entrails, the testes of hares — cocks — stags, semen from animals or humans, excrement, blood and brains of birds, animal secretions, urine, hummingbird hearts.

The poet Propertius refers to a formula containing snake bones, a toad and the feathers of a screech owl.

Apuleius the novelist, in the *Metamorphoses,* includes among other ingredients a skull torn from the teeth of a wild animal.

Among the Navajo Indians, cow ordure was used. The Apache treated human excrement as an erotic aid while, in Africa, the Hottentots describe the use of urine as an aid to human sexuality.

Horace describes a typical love potion composed by the witch Canidia:

Canidia crown'd with writhing snakes
Dishevell'd thus the silence breaks,
"Now the magic fire prepare,
And from the grave, uprooted tear
Trees, whose horrors gloomy spread
Round the mansions of the dead
Bring the eggs and plumage foul
Of a midnight shrieking owl,
Be they well besmear'd with blood
Of the blackest venom'd toad,
Bring the choicest drugs of Spain,
Produce of the poisonous plain,
Then into the charm be thrown,
Snatch'd from famish'd bitch, a bone,
Burn them all with magic flame,
Kindled first by Colchian dame."

Phoeniculum vulgare

Fennel

Tufts of fennel in wine are said to stir the seed into action.

Phoenix dactylifera

The date palm is a very nutritious fruit. The Arabs believe that an infusion of this fruit in milk is aphrodisiac in activity.

Phosphorus

Foods containing this element are considered to be aphrodisiacs.

Phosphorus has long been considered to be a powerful stimulant to the generative organs. Workers in plants which manufactured matches, when they were made of a phosphorus compound, walked around with constant erections. Some were so painful they had to leave their jobs at intervals and walk around in the outside air until their erections eased.

Phydslis alkekengi

Winter berry

The alkaloids and bitters found in this fruit, plus its large amount of vitamin C, help make it a sexual stimulant.

Physalis angulata

Ground cherry

In the northern part of Nigeria, this plant is used by women when they find a lack of enthusiasm for congress with their husbands.

Physalis minima

Cape gooseberry

The fruit is suggested to infuse a worn-out sexual system with new vigor.

In Guam, both the natives and chickens love the fruit. The chickens pluck the fruit from the shrub while the natives make a salad containing the gooseberry plus other raw produce.

Pimento

Although it is now thought of as a spice called allspice, in the 12th century it was forbidden to be eaten by monks due to the reputation it had of its ability to stimulate the genitals.

A poultice of pimento and peppers boiled together with mallow and applied to the penis was considered a sexual stimulant in China.

Pimpinella anisum

Anise

This herb was known to Dioscorides, ancient Greek botanist but it was not until the Middle Ages that it came to be valued as an aphrodisiac.

Ancient Romans prepared wedding cakes and cookies with anise seed to insure a pleasant wedding night.

Pineapple

Plain or mixed with meat or fowl, pineapple's tart taste was regarded as stimulating to the genitourinary tract.

Piper cubeba

Cubebs

This pepper has a reputation for aphrodisiacal activity among many peoples, particularly the Chinese and the Arabs. Among the Hindus, the dried berry is steeped in the wedding wine when the groom has passed his fortieth birthday.

Piper guineense

West African pepper

In this case it is the leaves that are used to improve relations. Chewed or soaked in wine, or added to salads, young leaves are most popular among the natives.

Pistacia vera

Pistachio

This nut is frequently mentioned in Arab erotic books as having erotic value. It is very nutritious, particularly to the female principle but the bark of the tree is valuable to males.

Pisteriona

Albertus Magnus, in his *De Secretis Mulierum*, states that this plant — also called Hierobota, increases the state of passion even when held in the hand.

Plantago major

Plantain

The seed promotes the production of semen.

Plover's Eggs

These eggs, when stuffed with a spice mixture, were a favorite arousal method of Madame duBarry. She called it a means to arouse irresistible amorous situations.

Plutarch

Greek philosopher of the first century A.D. He wrote *De Sanitate Tuenda Praecepta*, about the preservation of health in which he discusses diuretics and love potions.

Polignonia

Also known as Corrigiola, an herb whose juice is a potent aphrodisiac according to Magnus.

Pomegranate

According to Pliny the Elder, the pith of the fruit was conducive to sexual play.

Potato

In the seventeenth century, the potato was believed to possess definite aphrodisiac qualities.

Prawns

The aphrodisiac nature of prawns was popularized by the Greek poet Asclepeades who prepared a dinner with fish and prawns as a means of stimulating sexual desire.

Premna Spinosa

Hindu erotology recommends as provocative of amatory vigor, a drink composed of the following:

Pounded fruits of the premna spinosa plant, asparagus, and the shvadaustra plant boiled in water.

Provincia

Chaldean's called it *Iterisi,* Magnus said it is an aphrodisiac herb which worked on men or women when eaten with food.

Psoralea corylifolia

This plant is native to India and China. The seeds are aromatic and pungent in flavor and are regarded as being powerful stimulants and tonics to the genital organs. They have been prescribed for all sorts of sexual incompetency.

Pudenda Muliebria

Depilation of these organs was practiced in ancient times. It was common practice among the harems in Turkey and the object was to provoke the amatory inclinations of their partners.

Purslane

This is a salad herb usually found growing near water. Its reputation as an aphrodisiac appears to be unfounded since it is really anti-aphrodisiac in action.

Pyrethrum

Pyrethrum parthenium

The Greeks called it "the plant that kindles love." The Arabs pounded pyrethrum, ginger and lilac into an ointment that was used to massage the genital area as a prelude to a sexual encounter.

Q

Quince Jelly

Reputedly, this jelly has decided erotic effects. Possibly due to the bitter taste of the quince which acts upon the gastrourinary tract and the energy gained from the sugar.

Quinine

This bitter tasting alkaloid, which is used in modern times as a treatment for malaria, was used by the Ancient Persians as an aphrodisiac aid. The bark, which contains the alkaloid, was boiled to make a tea, then sweetened with honey and taken three times a day.

R

Radishes

Radishes, beans, peas, and lentils were considered to have a stimulating effect and were eaten as coital aids.

Rakta-Bol

The Hindu name for myrrh. Powdered myrrh, costus arabicus, manishil, borax and aniseed were mixed with sesame oil and gently massaged into the penis and scrotum.

Rejuvenation Recipe

A Hindu manual of love recommends a lotion made from juice of the roots of the madayantaka plant, yellow amaranth, anjanika plant, the clitoria ternateea, and the shlakshnaparni plant. Apply and couple!

Reptiles

All sorts of snakes were considered to have aphrodisiac abilities according to the ancient Romans. In the American West, rattlesnake meat had the same reputation.

Reserpine

An herbal drug used to reduce blood pressure that can also induce erotic dreams and have an aphrodisiac effect.

Although it was introduced into modern medicine about thirty years ago, it was used in India for thousands of years for all kinds of illnesses. The plant was called sarpagandha in Sanskrit which meant *insanity cure*. The dried root was chewed by holy men as an aid to relaxation.

Resin

All resins that oozed from plants and trees were considered to be stimulants according to the ancient Greeks and Romans.

Rhinoceros Horn

This is one aphrodisiac which causes great harm in the animal world since it is destroying a species of animal. The use of rhinoceros horn continues as you read this.

The horn is in great demand in India, China and Southeast Asia and no amount of medical proof is able to sway belief in this aphrodisiacal remedy. This belief holds that a love potion which contains rhino horn is able to change a tired penis into a formidable lance able to dip repeatedly into the honey pot.

The use of deer horn for the same purpose causes no such problems of destruction because the deer will shed its horns each year after the mating season is over. However, this practice with the rhinoceros's is threatening them with extinction.

Rhynchosia phaseolides

Pega palo

Wondrous virility powers are attributed to this vine found on the island of Haiti. One inch of the vine is steeped in a bottle of rum for seven days, after which doses are taken in a shot glass no more than two times a day. If too much is taken at one time, the result could be an arousal that wouldn't relax until it became so painful the owner had to support it in a sling.

The vine grows only on the hillsides and evidently enjoys alternate sun and shade. It has the appearance of an electric extension cord with three or four strands of the dark green vine twined about each other.

Pega palo can be found in some bars in Miami.

Rice

An effective sexual preparation, according to Hindu erotology is:

Mix sparrows' eggs (hens' eggs will do as well) and rice, boiled in milk, to which are added honey and ghee. Drink.

The *Ananga-Ranga* suggests wild rice mixed with honey of equal weights, eaten in the evening.

Rice Oil

Ruta graveolens

The fresh leaves of this plant yield a yellow oil which appears to have the irritating effects of cantharides with slightly less danger. The irritant action upon the genitalia may be construed as aphrodisiac in nature but its use is too dangerous when so many other effective methods are at hand.

Rivière

Exponent of the following formula used in the sixteenth century:

Amber, 1/2 dram
Musk, 2 scruples
Aloes, 1 dram
Pound together, then cover completely with spirits of wine.
Heat, filter, mix with:
Cinnamon water, 4 ounces
Orange water, 6 ounces
Rosewater, 6 ounces

Rocket

Brassica eruca

A kind of cabbage that is found in the Mediterranean. Used in salads by the natives of that region, it is reputed to have aphrodisiac qualities. Horace and Martial refer to its ability to arouse sexual interest in jaded individuals.

Rocket restores vigor to the genitals and was consecrated to Priapus.

Rocket Salad

Mix the cabbage with olive oil, vinegar, pepper and chopped garlic for an invigorating, salacious salad.

Roe

Cod and herring roe are considered high in aphrodisiac potential.

Rosa moschata

Musk-scent rose

This is a variety of rose noted for its ability to inspire an unrelenting desire for lovemaking. The scent, which remarkably resembles the odor of musk, is said to motivate amatory expression in exhausted males if there is still the slightest spark of life.

The rose is cultivated in India and an attar is prepared from its petals. Shop around in Indian stores until you find some.

Rubus species

Chinese raspberry

Dried raspberries are used in China to give vigor to the body and as an aphrodisiac.

Rue

Along with water lily, endive, and lettuce, rue was believed to have slightly stimulating qualities.

S

Safflower

A thistle-like plant recommended as a sexual stimulant in the fourth century.

Saffron

A Greek legend says that any girl eating saffron for a week could not resist a lover.

Saffron, except for tiny doses, can kill you!

A concoction of saffron, orange blossoms, dried dates, anise, wild carrots, and egg yolk, boiled in water into which honey and the blood of two freshly killed doves have been poured is recommended by Arabian erotic manuals as very aphrodisiac in action.

Saint Ignatius Bean

Strychnos ignatii

Grows in the Philippines and is a source of strychnine. Formerly thought of as an aphrodisiac because of its ability to improve rigidity . . . but the type of rigidity it promotes leads to death.

Leave this bean strictly alone.

Salep

Satyrion

A nymph and a satyr made love and their offspring was named Orchis. During a drunken revel to Bacchus, he approached one of the god's virgin priestesses who had had one cup too much of delicious wine, and — in a furious tussle — she was no longer a virgin. This outraged the other members of the party and they physically tore Orchis to pieces.

The satyr father, overcome with grief, begged the gods to reassemble his son. They thought the world was better off without the drunken lout but, moved by the father's pleas, they decreed that some of his parts could return to earth each spring as the flowers which bear his name — orchids!

So, that's the reason orchids have two bulbous roots, each shaped like an *orchis* (Greek for testicle), and the reputation as the ultimate aphrodisiac.

Theophrastus, in his book, *Enquiry into Plants,* tells of an orchid sent to Antiochus, King of Syria, that was so potent the delivery man was able to have sex with seventy women in a row, stopping only when his member was so wounded that it pained him too much to make an entrance.

And he had just held the plant in his hands!

Hercules was able to repay the hospitality of Thespius by deflowering his fifty virgin daughters after one drink of orchis.

The English concocted a mixture of orchis boiled in muscatel, with chestnuts, pistachios, pine nuts, cubeb, peppers, cinnamon, rocket seed, and sugar.

Gradually, the name satyrion was replaced by salep, borrowed from the Arabic *sahlap* from "testicles of the fox."

What made orchis so powerful?

It does contain a starchlike substance called bassorin which energizes the body, tones the muscles, and serves as a complex-carbohydrate food source. Perhaps there is some hidden ingredient not discovered by science. The Zulu in Africa chew the root of orchis and consider it to be a potent aphrodisiac to this day. So . . . give it a try.

Salvadore oleoides

Mustard tree

The fruit of the tree is said to arouse a tired member, but can cause sores in the mouth. Better to use the shoots and young leaves with a meal of chicken and onions.

Salvia

Sage

The genus of plant that is used as a garnish and also has a reputation as an aphrodisiac.

Salvia haematodes

Bloody sage

The root is the source of a bitter alkaloid largely prescribed for seminal debility in India.

Salvia officinalis

Garden sage

Sage was thought to assist fertility. It is widely used for its taste and aroma in cooking. The pungent taste helps digest meals containing meat.

Salvia plebia

East Indian sage

The seeds of this variety are used for seminal weakness and to promote sexual awareness.

Salvia sclarea

Clary sage

The seeds are powdered and mixed with wine to insure a lusty desire for sexual union.

Samayamatrika

An Indian erotic manual by Kshemendra which is similar in content and intent to the *Kama Sutra*.

Sandix ceropolium

Tiberius, Emperor of Rome, used this plant because of its reputation for exciting amorous propensities.

Sanseviera

A Hindu formula for sexual stimulus is made from the seeds of the sanseviera roxburghiana, long pepper, and the seeds of Hedysarum gangeticum, ground together and mixed with warm milk.

Santonin

This is extracted from the dried flower heads of the plant called Artemisia maritima and used to be called an aphrodisiac. However, instead it can cause poisoning, followed by coma and death. So stay away except for medicinal use when prescribed by a physician.

Sarsaparilla

The Indians used it as a blood fortifier and to treat impotence. In the 1500's, a Spanish doctor named Monardes studied the plant and introduced it into "accepted" medicine.

In 1939, a Hungarian chemist named Solmo, working in Mexico, discovered that the bark of the Smilax aristalochiafolia (sarsaparilla) contained sterones. Testosterone is essential in the male to restore a fully developed penis, a beard, and all other male attributes, including whistle-provoking muscles as well. It's found naturally in the bark of this tree.

It's not only important to the male of the species because females also need testosterone for their sexual drive to mature. But nature thought of the female when it grew this plant. Sarsaparilla also contains sarsapogenin for making the female hormone that helps defend us against infection.

Not bad for a simple plant the Indians knew about for centuries.

Sarsaparilla tea, in which the root bark is prepared in water, is really too weak to be considered a real aphrodisiac, but here's a recipe that will do very well in most cases of lax libido caused by hormonal insufficiency:

Take 2 heaping teaspoons of shaved, inner root bark (about 1/4 ounce) and let simmer in 1 pint of water for about ten minutes. There will be a lot of foam due to the saponins in the bark so watch that it doesn't boil over. This method differs from tea-making in that the material is heated for ten minutes instead of merely standing in hot water.

Drink up to 2 cups of this mixture morning and night, holding the fluid in the mouth so the sterones can be absorbed through the mucous membrane of the mouth, then swallow.

Or, if you've a mind to make the tincture of sarsaparilla, get a bottle and fill it half full of bark. Then add half water and half vodka to fill the bottle. Let stand for two weeks making sure to shake the bottle daily. At the end of the time, filter and take a tablespoon of the liquid 3 or 4 times a day.

Don't make a habit of taking this herbal. Just long enough to restore what was lost to you, then discontinue it. You want your body to make its own hormones and not depend on a drink.

Satureja hortensis

Summer savory

An infusion of this herb is warming to the stomach and the genitals.

Satyriasis

A condition of intense and excessive sexual involvement. Usually associated with a satyr — half goat and half human — attendant of the God Pan. Their unbridled lustfulness was part and parcel of their being.

Saussurea lappa

Costus

In the Malay peninsula the root is considered to be a sexual tonic. Many of the peoples of the East judge a tonic by its aphrodisiac ability. The alkaloid saussurine is present in greatest amounts in the root during the months of September and October and the best medicinal roots are gathered in those months.

The plant also contains an essential oil which is excreted mainly in the urine. Its passage through the genitourinary tract may be the cause of the aphrodisiacal effects.

Sauterne

This wine is believed by some to be able to excite an amorous adventure providing it is taken in small amounts. Large amounts tend to make one sleepy and unable to perform.

Saw Palmetto

Serenoa serrulata

This plant grows in the U.S. and has sweet reddish-brown to purple berries that look a lot like dark olives. They are popular among herbalists for building up muscle and glandular tissue.

They have also been used in cases where sperm production is low. Also, it is claimed that long-term use can develop breasts that have not reached the dimensions the owner has hoped for.

The berries, especially when fresh, are one of the safest and most beneficial of the aphrodisiacs. Eat a dozen a day. If only the dried berries are available you can eat them as is, reconstitute them in water, or powder them and make a tea.

Most health food stores or herbal stores will carry the dried variety. If you live within five miles of the Atlantic shore from Florida to South Carolina, you may be able to gather them for yourself. Make sure they are Saw Palmetto berries before eating them.

Scammony

This is a gummy resin exudate used as a medicine in the Middle East. Avicenna recommends that it be combined with honey and taken daily as an aphrodisiac.

Scrophularia oldhami

Figwort

The root is dried until it becomes a black-purple in color. That's when it is at its sweetest and most potent.

Sea Foods

All seafood, fish, shellfish, bivalves, etc. have the reputation for being aphrodisiacs. This may be because they are highly nutritious and easily digestible. But, they also contain many sea minerals such as phosphorus and iodine which do influence the sensual being.

Octopus and cuttlefish, as well as caviar, are also reputed to be of value in this arena. In the Orient, shark fin soup is much esteemed as a food and an aphrodisiac. In parts of Europe, the eel is believed to give the penis strength. The West Indies believe that the conch provides penile power. Sea turtle eggs and sea urchin provide Barbadians with virility.

Sea Slug

The West Indies is the natural home for this ocean resident. In Italy it is called sea proapus because of its reputation for raising an erection when all else has failed.

Semecarpus anacardium

Oriental Cashew

In India, this fruit is said to keep old men free from colds and senile degeneration.

Sensitive Plant

Mimosa pudica

In the Amazon basin, some tribes take the roots of this plant and squeeze the juice from it. Then they take the leaves and soak them in the juice. The resultant is then painted on their breasts to give them greater sexual stamina and more orgasms.

You can do the same. The plant is a household plant called touch-me-not that might be growing in your window box. Can she absorb its mysterious ingredients by your simply painting her breasts? Why not? LSD 25 can affect you simply by being applied to the skin.

In the case of mimosa, it does contain psychedelic components called tryptamines.

Certain Peruvian tribes make use of the mimosa by chewing on the leaves and the root.

Sesame Stimulant

Mix the outer husk of the sesame seed with sparrows' eggs, milk, sugar, ghee and honey. Add beans and wheat flour, and the fruit of the trapa bispinosa. Mix well and take daily until the impulse to make love rejoins your tired body.

Sesamum orientale

A decoction of the seed ground up with linseed is used in the Philippines as an aphrodisiac.

Sesame has been cultivated since ancient times. The leaves are steeped in hot water as a tea, the oil is used in cooking and on salads as well as on the skin as a softening agent. Taken internally in quantity, it has a laxative effect. In August of 1990, it was reported as a cure for warts in East-West Magazine.

Sesame seeds are very nutritious and eating them will nourish all parts of the body including the procreative ones.

Shallot

A small onion much desired in making sauces. If age relaxes the nuptial knot, thy food be onions and thy feast shallot.

Sheep

Think of this on your wedding night. In ancient Persia, sheep testicles steeped in vinegar were considered a sexual inducement.

Shorea robusta

Dammar resin tree

When the stem is bruised it exudes an oleo-resin gum with an aromatic odor that is said to stimulate sexual desire. The resin is gathered in the morning, then fried in ghee and strained through water to clarify it. The thicker layer contains the aphrodisiac elements.

Shunga

Japanese erotic wood block prints. The artists went into great detail and these prints are prized as being among the most erotic and most beautiful renditions of sexual union extant.

Sida cordifolia

Although the entire plant carries the alkaloid ephedra, a central nervous system stimulant, the seeds have the highest concentration. Because of their stimulant action they are used as an aphrodisiac, particularly in India.

Silphium perfoliatum

Indian cup-plant

In India, it is said that this plant makes an old man young. It is used as a strong decoction. Brew the root for twenty minutes.

Skink

Scincus officinalis.

A small lizard found in North Africa and Arabia. Prized medicinally and thought of as an aphrodisiac when fried in oil.

Snails

The Roman poets of yesteryear referred to them as potent aphrodisiacs. This is a recipe from an old volume of erotic cookery:

Boil snails with onions, parsley and garlic. Then drain and fry the mixture in olive oil. After that, remove from the oil and boil again in red wine.

Have this recipe for dinner on the night you wish to enjoy the love of a woman.

Snuff

According to *The Perfumed Garden*, snuff, plain or perfumed, can act as a sexual stimulant.

Solanum indicum

Indian nightshade

The root is macerated in alcohol, strained and made into a strong drink that is exciting to the animal nature.

Solanum melongena

Egg plant

Not to be confused with eggplant. In Africa it is used as an aphrodisiac by extracting the juice, but in Nigeria it is taken by women to insure fertility.

Solanum nigrum

Black nightshade

The younger shoots are plucked, blanched in boiling water and eaten by men and women. The men say it increases sexual ability while the women say it helps relieve menstrual problems.

Song of Nala

An epic Hindu poem of magic devices, spells, incantations and potions to stimulate sexual potency. One of the stories is of King Brihadratha, ruler of Magadha, who wanted a son but, although steeped in sexual pleasures, was unable to sire an heir.

He consulted a seer who advised him to stand under a mango tree and take the first ripe mango that falls near him and give it to his favorite wife. He had two favorites so he cut the fruit in half and gave half to each. Sure enough, each got pregnant and presented him with half a son. However, through magical intervention the two parts were joined together and he finally had a male heir.

Soup

Fish soup is considered to be an aphrodisiac in character. Among stimulating soups are onion soup, cheese soup, lentil soup, mushroom soup, celery soup.

Southernwood

Historia naturalis

According to Pliny the Elder, southernwood was conducive to sexual excitement and you didn't even have to make it into a tea or soup. Simply place the wood under the bed.

Sparrows

Male sparrows fried in olive oil were considered a treat to heighten sexual pleasure.

Sphaeranthus hirtus

Indian thistle

The root is steeped in warm water for twelve hours after which it is boiled in sesame water. The resulting mix is to be taken first thing in the morning on an empty stomach for one month in a dose of 2 drams. The effect is strongly aphrodisiac.

Spinach

Was often considered an amatory stimulant because of its nutritional content.

Spondias amara

In this case it is the fruit that is thought to be favorable to sexual skill and performance.

Spurge

The milky juice plus cardamon, cinnamon, pellitory, ginger and nettle seed is an Arabic specific for sexual weakness.

Storgethron

The ancient Greeks thought of this plant as a love medicine. It has been identified as the common leek.

Stramonium

Datura stramonium

The seed mixed in wine produces libidinous activity. Excessive consumption can lead to hallucinations and death.

Sturgeon Soup

Considered to be rich in aphrodisiac elements, this fish soup is popular in the Mediterranean area.

Swallow Nest Soup

Popular in China for restoring exhausted potency.

Swan

Swan's genitals have been used in erotic cookery as an aphrodisiac.

Sexual Activity

Arnold Lorand, M.D., wrote in his book, "*The Increase of Sexual Activity by a Specially Altered Diet,*" that since the most remote periods of the existence of man, the eating of fish and fish parts has been accredited with the property of increasing sexual activity. It is for this reason that the ancient Egyptians forbade the eating of fish by their priests.

William J. Robinson, M.D., wrote in his book, "*America's Sex and Marriage Problems,*" that caviar is the treatment of choice in cases of nutritionally reversible impotence.

So, to paraphrase Marie, "let them eat fish."

T

Tacca involucrata

In Africa, the tubers of this plant were considered to be stimulating in nature and were so powerful that they were reserved only for the ruling class.

Tapirs

The meat was considered to be a feast but the hoofs were used as a sexual stimulant.

The male tapir's hoofs were scraped and mixed with native brew as an aphrodisiac. The female tapir's hoofs were used by women for fertility and sexual enjoyment. Great care was taken that the scraping should not be mixed because great harm would come to a man who took a female tapir's hoof.

Tarragon

The leaves of this plant are used to flavor salads and other foods, but the root, powdered and served with wine is said to be a sexual stimulant.

Testes

Animal testicles were assumed to possess powerful sexual virtues. Alexander Dumas, a master chef, as well as a writer of considerable skill, recommended the balls of the ram with mushrooms, onions and garlic, sautéed in wine.

In France, Mme. de Pompadour was served such a dish by Louis XV as an inducement to sexual dalliance.

In Arabia and Morocco, lion's testicles are considered to be best for this purpose.

Many aphrodisiac recipes rely on the ass to contribute its testicles.

Testicular Application

In the second century A.D., Galen, the Greek physician, considered that applications of special combinations of substances to the genitals were erotically stimulating. One such mixture is as follows:

> *Cinnamon powder, gilliflower, ginger, rose wine, theriac, rosewater and breadcrumbs.*

Tetragastris balsamifera

Bois cochon

This tree is native to Haiti. The outer and inner bark is steeped in warm water for several days, then strained and the liquid portion is used as an aphrodisiac.

If there is no response to the first treatment, the bark is then mixed with leane bande (Rhynchosia) before steeping.

Thyme

This fragrant herb is used as a spice, for medicinal purposes, and as a sexual stimulant.

Tinospora cordifolia

Moonseed

This plant is a creeping vine and the fresher it is, the more powerful is its action as an aphrodisiac. All parts of the plant are used but the roots are considered to be nutritive as well as stimulating.

Tonka

Coumaraouna odorata

The ripe seeds of this plant have been used as an aphrodisiac but newer investigations consider the extract to be poisonous. The use of this herbal is not worth the risk. Stay away from any form of tonka beans. They have a fragrant aroma and a bitter taste and are sometimes used to make necklaces.

Tortilis japonica

Hedge parsley

Provokes erection of the parts is the word about his herbal.

Trapa Bispinosa

A plant used in Hindu love potions in the following manner:

Take the roots or the seeds of the plants Trapa bispinosa, tuscan jasmine, kasurika, and licorice and powder them. Add the bulbous portion of the plant called kshirika, mix with sugar, milk and ghee, boil for fifteen minutes and drink.

Tribulus terrestris

Caltrope

The plant, fruit and roots are made into an infusion and served with rice to rebuild a tired sexual libido into a robust young thrusting member.

Trigonella foenum graecum

Fenugreek

A decoction of seeds flavored with mint or lemon is used in Germany, Hungary and Austria as an aid to sexual congress. Fenugreek is very nourishing and is a source of energy to the entire body. It can be made into a tea.

Truffle

An edible fungus indigenous to Europe and known to the Ancient Romans as a powerful stimulant to lovemaking. Napoleon used to eat truffles to increase his potency after being advised by one of his generals of its power.

Turnips

Turnips stewed in milk have a reputation as being very helpful in cases of diminished potency.

U

Uchata

A mixture of the roots of the uchata, piper cubeba and Chinese licorice, mixed with sugar and milk make a beverage which, in Hindu erotic circles, influences a positive sexual reaction.

Urid

In the *Anaga-Ranga,* the recipe for amatory assertiveness is as follows:

Steep urid seeds in milk and sugar. Leave the mixture in the sun for three days or until the milk evaporates. Take what is left and knead it into cakes which are then fried in ghee. Eat one cake each morning for seven days.

Urtica dioica

Stinging nettle

Crush the fresh seed in wine to promote warm feelings.

V

Valerian

This herb has been used for "woman's troubles" for hundreds of years in spite of its odor, and is very effective. And this finding still remains unexplained: it has also been used to stimulate affection so even when she is not particularly fond of you, she can't resist lavishing you with physical affection.

Vanilla planifolia

Vanilla

Vanilla is actually an orchid. It is one of the most popular of all flavors and has had a reputation as an aphrodisiac for centuries. Whether swallowed or applied to the genitals, it has been an exciting, sensual aid since first being discovered.

Vanilla

According to Corneille de Blessbois (*Venus en Rut*), vanilla turned most men on. Madame de Pompadour preferred to mix chocolate with vanilla and a drop of amber. If that failed to arouse the amorous spark, truffles sliced into celery soup turned ordinary into extraordinary.

Veal Sweetbread

There appears to be some sexual connection between this dish and a lazy lover. Worth a try.

Venison

Along with other meat, it is thought of as sexually stimulating.

Verbascum thapsus

Mullein

The leaves, flowers, seeds and root are considered to be sexual stimulants. In India, the ground seed is mixed with warmed milk and sugar and taken late in the evening as a sexual aid.

Veronia amygdalina

Bitter leaf

Boil the young leaves through several changes of water and then mix them with sweetened butter to make yourself more sexually attractive to the opposite sex. This may be the most unbelievable manifestation of all, till you document its effects again and again.

Vinca major

Periwinkle

An antibiotic was recently discovered in the sap of this plant but it has been used to promote sexual appetite for centuries.

Albertus Magnus recommended it combined with earth worms and an herb called Sempervivum tectorium to induce love.

Vinca rosea

Pink periwinkle

In Haiti, an infusion is used to lower the sugar content of the blood, therefore it is considered to be an aid to those with diabetes. Gypsies considered it to be an aid to lust.

Vitamins

(See also Appendix, page 311)

Foods affect our moods. Vitamins, in particular, can affect our sex life. This is a brief rundown on the individual vitamins and what they do, in part, to keep you sexually up!

Vitamin A

This vitamin cannot be manufactured in the body and is necessary for normal reproduction. If there is a lack of vitamin A, the testes and the ovaries of male and female rats atrophy . . . so who is to say that the same thing cannot happen in people. In male rats, sperm formation declines drastically. In both male and female, sex hormone production is impaired.

Physically, the mucous membrane of the vagina depends on vitamin A for healthy lubrication. Without it the membrane becomes dry, cracked and painful. Who can think about sex when every touch is painful?

B-Complex Family

Vitamin B^1 is essential to energy production. A lack of this vitamin can drain your energy and put an end to your sex life.

Vitamin B^2 is also involved in energy production. Any lack of any B-vitamins will drain your resources.

Vitamin B^3 (niacin) enhances your sexual ability by dilating blood vessels and stimulating circulation to the extremities.

If there is a lack of vitamin B^6, you can lose your sex drive entirely.

Pantothenic Acid. This vitamin, one of the B's, helps to make steroid hormones and choline which are necessary for sexual arousal.

Inositol is needed by the brain and the sexual arousal system.

Vitamin C

Will affect the sex life directly through its role in the absorption of iron, the formation of red blood, and the health of the adrenal glands. All of the processes have an influence on your sex life. The adrenal glands make several hormones and neurotransmitters that exert power on your sex life including one involved in stimulating orgasm.

Vitamin E

The hormones you need to make sex depend on vitamin E to protect them from oxidation. Vitamin E also increases your energy capacity.

All vitamins are important to you. Some can be found in foods and others must be supplemented in order that the necessary amounts be available when your body demands them.

Vulvae Steriles

The vulvae of the sow were popular as a gourmet's dish and credited with erotic effects.

W

Water Lily

This will work against any desire for sex according to a church decree that all monks and nuns should drink a mixture of water lilies and syrup of poppies. It would appear that the poppies alone would do the trick!

White Wine

Mix with juniper berries, quassia, and bitter orange syrup. Drink for the proper amatory direction.

Whiting

Like most fish, whiting is considered nourishing and stimulating to desire.

Winged Ant

Used in place of Spanish Fly during the Renaissance.

Witch-Hazel

Externally applied to the genitalia, witch-hazel allows an indomitable tower of potency that lasts beyond climax after climax.

Red Wine Please!

Red wine is said to promote relaxation and a lessening of inhibitions.

It has been said through the ages that red wine is an aphrodisiac and, according to modern medical science, it may be true.

Red wine causes the body to produce histamines.

Pharmaceutical experiments indicate that histamines can shorten the time between arousal and satisfaction . . . and intensify the experience.

Women benefit from drinking red wine more than men.

That should be obvious!

Woodcock

This bird makes a delightful meal and is reputed to stimulate the production of seminal fluid.

Withania somnifera

Winter cherry

The root of this herb contains an alkaloid called somniferine which is a powerful aphrodisiac. 1/2 dram of the powdered root mixed with milk is the recommended dose.

Wrightia tinctoria

Sweet indrajac

The seeds, smashed and mixed with sour wine, are used in India for seminal weakness.

X

Xylopia aethiopica

Spice tree

To encourage fertility, use a decoction of the fruit or the bark.

Asparagus and Beets

Pliny speaks of asparagus and white beets as useful to arousal while in parts of Germany the men eat flatulent foods like beans, peas, lentils and radishes in order to obtain more powerful parts by way of the accumulated gas.

Y

Yarrow

Medieval witches prepared a potion for newly-married couples to insure seven years of sexy living. Yarrow was one of the ingredients.

Yohimbine

Stimulates the nerves of the spinal column which stimulate the genitalia (See also "Yohimbine", page 42).

Aphrodisiac Dinner

Aphrodisiac Dinner as prepared for the Marquis de Sade in his *120 Journées de Sodome*: bisque, twenty hors d'oeuvres, twenty entrées, poultry, game garnished and shaped fantastically, roasts, pastries — hot and cold — dessert, fruits, ices, chocolates, liqueurs, Burgundy, Rhone and Rhine wines and champagne.

A plenteous meal may produce voluptuous sensations (*le bon diner peut causer une volupté physique*).

Z

Zanthoxylum rhetsa

Used in India and Ceylon. The fruit is used as a condiment in curries but the bark is thought to be an aphrodisiac.

Casanova

Casanova was born in 1725 and died in 1798. He died in the company of three women doing what he did best to the last. Next to the bed, in a royal purple vase, was a mysterious liquid. Casanova would frequently drink of this liquid, offering wine to his guests instead.

Was this the secret to his bedroom prowess, the key to how he was able to bed more than one woman at a time?

Although analysis was not as good in the 1700's as today, some enterprising fellow made off with the vase after his death. He took it to the chemist and they believe this was the formula:

Casanova's Cocktail

1/2 cup fresh grapefruit juice
1/2 cup steamed apple juice
1/2 teaspoonful of cinnamon powder

Mix vigorously, then sip.

Was there a secret ingredient the chemist failed to find? Or did he find it and merely give this formula to the thief? There are rumors that a chemist became the greatest lover in Italy after the death of Casanova. Could it have been the chemist who had a shot at this famous elixir of love?

Cleopatra

First Julius fell to her charms and then it was Marc Antony's turn. What was it about Cleopatra that made men fall at her feet — then into her boudoir? Legend has it that she would prepare a potion for her lovers that promoted "unendurable pleasure, indefinitely prolonged."

However, it was not a potion for her lovers alone. She also would partake of the mixture and meet each demand with a counter-demand of her own. Although well into her fourth decade, she performed with the vigor and sexual response of an adolescent.

What was this mystical brew that made men greater lovers than they had ever been? A special maid would put together the following mixture. It had to be mixed vigorously and, after mixing, was shaken for 10 minutes by a robust Nubian slave who enjoyed the confidence of his mistress.

Nowadays we have a blender that can do the job more quickly.

Cleopatra's Elixir of Everlasting Love

In a blender place:

1/4 cup bananas, squashed thoroughly
1/4 cup watermelon juice, no seeds
1/2 cup unripe papaya juice
1/2 teaspoonful powdered cloves

Blend at high speed until thoroughly mixed.
Sip slowly before engaging in a carnal cuddle.

Farfetched?

Not nutritionally speaking, since the combination of minerals, protein, vitamins in the fruit, plus the natural ingredients in the cloves combine to produce a stimulant to the sex glands and hormones. Experts have told us that Cleopatra would frequently go on a 24-hour fast existing solely on this potion and no other food. Then the Queen of the Nile would reemerge from her boudoir to give and receive another 24-hour pleasure trip.

The Erotology Of Food

Albertus Magnus

The brains of a partridge calcined into powder and swallowed with red wine.

Platina

The flesh of the partridge, which is of good and easy digestion, is highly nutritious; it strengthens the brain, facilitates conception and arouses the half-extinct desire for venereal pleasures.

From *De Valetudine Tuenda*

Mery

For the purpose, the *partes genitales* of a cock prepared in wine.

From *Traité Universel des Drogues Simples.*

Aqua Magnaanitatis

Take of ants a handful of their eggs, two hundred wood lice, two hundred of bees, into a jar with spirits. Digest them a month, then pour off the clear spirits and drink thus with the flesh of fowl.

Juvenal

The mollusca in general, and testaceous animals in particular, have been considered as endowed with aphrodisiac properties. Oysters and mussels have in this respect become vulgarly proverbial.

For what cares the drunken dame (take head or tail), to her 'tis much the same
Who at deep midnight on fat oysters sups.

Apuleius

Author of the *Golden Ass* writes of shellfish, lobster, sea hedgehogs, spiced oysters and cuttlefish, the last of which was particularly famed for its stimulating qualities.

This peculiar property has been attributed to the presence of phosphorus, which is known to exist somewhat plentifully in the substance, and has also been discovered in their roe in a simple state of combination.

Now, phosphorus is one of the most powerful stimulants: it acts upon the generative principles and organs in a manner to cause the most violent priapisms: but this principle does not act alone, and there must be taken into account the different seasonings and condiments which form the basis of most culinary preparations to which fish are subjected, and which are all taken from the class of irritants.

From *Hecquet* — 1709

A drake belonging to a chemist, having drunk water out of a copper vessel which had contained phosphorus, ceased not gallanting his females until he died.

An old man to whom a few drops only of phosphorus had been administered, experienced repeated and imperious venereal wants which he was compelled to satisfy.

From Seward — *Sex and the Social Order*, Pelican Books, 1954

Sensations of the same kind are said to be experienced by persons whose occupation requires handling of phosphorus. It may thus be considered as satisfactorily proved that the substance, derived from food or otherwise, is essentially a stimulant of the genital organs.

However, the administration of it, even in small doses, has been productive of the most horrible and fatal results! Phosphorus, as a chemical, is one of the most poisonous substances known to man and should never be used in supplemental form.

From Boswell — *Dissertatio Inaugaurilis de Ambra*

Three grains of ambergris in white wine will produce a marked acceleration of the pulse, a considerable development of muscular strength, a greater activity of the intellectual faculties, and a disposition to venereal desires.

The flesh of the lizard, particularly of the crocodile when taken near his genital organs, when cooked in sweet wine will cause an erection of the virile member.

From *Aelius Tetrabilis*

From: The Perfumed Garden

- *Take the fruit of the mastis tree, macerated well with oil and honey, drink of the liquid first thing in the morning and evening.*
- *Drink before going to bed a glassful of very thick honey and eat twenty almonds and one hundred pine nuts. Do this for three days, then pound onion seed mixed well with honey and take of this mixture while fasting.*
- *Green peas, boiled with onion, and then powdered with cinnamon, ginger and cardamom, create strength for coitus.*
- *Pastry containing honey, ginger, syrup of vinegar, hellebore, garlic, cinnamon, nutmeg, cardamom, sparrow's tongues, Chinese cinnamon, and long pepper.*
- *He who boils asparagus stalks, and then fries them in fat, and then pours upon them the yolks of eggs with pounded condiments and fries the mixture, then eats daily of this dish will find it stimulating for amorous desires.*
- *He who peels onions, puts them in a saucepan, with condiments and aromatic substances, and fries the mixture with oil and yolks of eggs, will acquire a surpassing and invaluable vigour.*
- *Camel's milk mixed with honey and taken regularly causes the virile member to be on the alert night and day.*

- *He who for several days makes his meals upon eggs boiled with myrrh, coarse cinnamon, and pepper, will find his vigour greatly increased.*

- *Take cubebs into the mouth with honey, scammony, ginger and pepper. Mix it thoroughly with your own saliva. Then apply it to the head of your penis. After a few applications, it will noticeably increase in size, but may be irritating although the increase in size may cause pleasure to your mate.*

- *To re-awaken juvenile ardor, the judicious use of fish soup, milk, ghee, garlic, onions and honey.*

PART TWO

THE LOVER'S COOKBOOK

Pasta Makes You Sleepy
Chewing On Salad Makes You Tired
Fiber Keeps You Regular . . .
But
That's Not What This Book Is About!
Sex Begins In The Kitchen,
Simmers At The Table,
Explodes In The Bedroom . . .
The Recipes In This Part Are Designed
To Stimulate The Libido,
Excite Your More Primitive Desires,
And Promote More And Better Sexual Congress!

Preface

There is a sad story about most marriages. It goes this way:

> *If you put a bean in a jar each time you make love the first two years of your marriage, and take a bean from the jar every time you make love after that . . . you will never take all of the beans out of the bottle.*

It is a sad story.

But it doesn't have to be your story.

Why?

Because of nutritional magic. Because sex begins in the mind and filters downwards.

This cookbook is different. It's about the smells and tastes of food and the hidden components that can tilt the mind toward thoughts of lovemaking, pleasure and excitement. It mixes the latest knowledge of food chemistry with the coarse understanding of sensuality that made certain chefs and certain women famous.

The feelings derived from food combinations can be manipulated by the knowing chef or knowing woman into the intense feeling of the bedroom. Verbal communication between husband and wife is still in its infancy but the communication of flavor, fragrance and phytochemicals (natural chemicals found in certain foods) is centuries old. Although people are different and their ability to taste and smell vary, all people respond to food chemistry in varying degrees.

How and what you cook, how and what you use to flavor your dishes can increase your shared pleasures, unleash hidden drives, and revive the excitement of your honeymoon.

Read this book for the best of your life!

Duc de Richelieu

The Duc de Richelieu, a nobleman with a reputation that vied with Casanova's, may have gone the final step. Not only did he search out the most potent of menus served to all of his friends and their mistresses, but all people at the dinner, including the servants, were completely naked.

Francis I

This sixteenth century king of France was known for his cultivated taste and amatory adventures. The latter was promoted by aphrodisiac foods and drink, particularly carp, lobster, caviar, eel, mullet, tuna, herring, mackerel, whiting and halibut.

Francis was noted for the number of his mistresses and died, some say, exhausted by excesses.

Foreplay

According to *The Perfumed Garden For The Soul's Delectation*, by Sheik Nefzawi who lived in the fifteenth century and who created the aphrodisiac-of-the-month club, the world's first erotic cookbook, there were eight essentials for sexual delight. Good nourishment led the list.

The art of cookery — and it is an art — has filled more books than any other subject except religion. Food and lovemaking have been intertwined, whether at a quiet dinner for two or an orgy for hundreds. Eat first is invisibly printed on every menu.

Cookbooks are those fundamental works which can be found in most homes as often as the Bible and the almanac. The cookbook, as a present to the bride, outranks every other gift in numbers and, as a restimulant to happier years, is now the number one anniversary gift.

It has been said that a woman's way to the heart of her man is through his stomach. This cliché, which is as old as Methuselah and found in the language of every nation, has its true origin in aphrodisiac cookery. From the oldest recorded history down to present times, those engaged in the preparation of food have passed along the knowledge that among all available foods, certain ones, certain condiments and beverages had a stimulating effect on those certain centers in our body which control our love lives.

Until recently, those recipes were hidden in the folklore and cookbooks of various nations. They were tried, found to be reasonably effective, and passed on. Nobody was interested in why!

That is, until now.

Modern science, sticking its nose into diet and nutrition, is beginning to unravel the why and wherefore of erotic cookery and beginning to substantiate some of the claims previously only whispered about from grandma's mouth to daughter's ear!

There are centers in the brain, everybody's brain, which can be stimulated by various substances naturally present in food. We only have to understand which foods do what in order to tilt the sexual attitude to a more loving inclination.

Is there a need for this stimulating cookery section?

You don't need statistically documented, expensive, long-term investigations into the marriage situation to discover that the largest percentage of unhappy marriages can be traced to the marriage bed. Outside pressures have become so predominant in the modern living environment that they almost exclude thoughts of lovemaking.

Our most wonderful emotion, most complete sharing of ourselves with another has been relegated to some secondary or tertiary position behind business or career or making money. All the T.V. and film advertising notwithstanding, the happiness of union is seriously lacking.

There are very few homes where, after the initial blush is off the rose, the wife does not wish for a greater show of affection and coupling than she is receiving from her previously passionate lover who is now merely her spouse.

Shouldn't it become obvious that uncovering the ways and means of restimulating affection via the legitimate route of cookery is an applaudable venture?

What better recommendation than that this cookery compilation should prove beneficial in that direction. That the preoccupied, not interested, grumpy individual sitting on the sofa in front of the T.V. should be restored to that ardent, passionate man you fell in love with.

Cookbooks are usually written by famous chefs, some of whom are gargantuan in size, interested only in satisfying the stomach. We are after lower satisfactions!

We have gathered together famous historical recipes which have proved to be worthwhile or they would have been forgotten. They have been brought up-to-date to conform to modern nutritional concepts. We have eliminated unhealthy practices such as too much salt or sugar, too much saturated fat. We've substituted olive oil or canola oil for lard and low-fat milk for whole milk. All of the recipes have been tested on one point. They make delicious dishes and do not contain any harmful substances.

Many of the recipes would be at home in any cookbook and, undoubtedly, millions of dinners have been consumed in which nobody was aware that the extraordinary satisfaction and increased desire was due to the preparation of the meal.

And why should it be announced?

Love is elusive and the love centers in the mind are fragile and resistant to manipulation if they're aware it is going on.

So don't tell. Use these recipes only as often as you wish to invite romance. After all, perhaps a constant diet of love can be tiring!

This is not a guide to gluttony but a gentle director to anticipatory epicurism.

Everyone Who Makes Love Believes in Aphrodisiacs!

People don't consciously think about it, but we all have something that sets us up for lovemaking. A favorite scent, an after-shave lotion, apple pie or maybe spiked heels.

Ovid states, "the best aphrodisiac is your own passion," but along with that he recommends a diet that includes honey, pine nuts, eggs, scallions, onions and basil.

Indians and Arabs thought that passion could be induced. They agreed on the fundamentals of milk and honey, onions and garlic, nuts and legumes, eggs, meat and a vast array of hot spices.

Sir Charles Carrinton, in 1900, translated Dr. Nicolas Venette's *Conjugal Love,* which praises seminal nutrifiers such as eggs, crabs, prawns, crayfish, beef marrow, milk, wine, vegetables which tend to cause wind, and cock testicles.

"Hot foods" were recommended in France: truffles, fish, mushrooms, asparagus, turtle soup, sweetbreads, shrimp and celery soup . . . all to lift the royal scepter.

Let's Keep Lovemaking At Home Where It Belongs

You Say That What I Cook Can Affect My Love Life?

Sure.

How Can That Be?

Well, you know how comfortably tired and relaxed you feel after a nice meal of pasta with mushrooms and a delicious sauce?

Yeah, Cozy And Sleepy.

That's because of the effect that the carbohydrates in the pasta have on your body chemistry. Sex begins in the brain and, if your brain is nice and sleepy, all relaxed, the inclination is to sleep . . . not to make love!

The brain is a chemical factory and the kinds of chemicals it manufactures depend on the food you give it. The brain talks to itself by means of chemical messengers called neurotransmitters. These internal messages influence your mood, your thoughts, your behavior, and your sex life.

If you want the messengers to play Cupid in your mate's head, you swing the thoughts to those of love by tilting to the production of the "right" chemical communication.

Pasta leads the brain to produce neurotransmitters called *serotonin*. These messengers tell the body to relax.

Isn't That Good?

Sure, if you're thinking of sleep and rest and a calm mind. But sex is strength, aggression, tension, desire . . . get the picture?

How Can That Come From My Menu?

It can't always come from the menu, it's not witchcraft! All you're doing is planting the right food so that, if all else is equal, natural events have a better chance.

When the chemical messengers being manufactured are *noradrenaline* and *dopamine,* you are conditioning the brain and mind toward the kind of behavior that can lead to the bedroom. The recipes in this book help to build the sexual appetite while they satisfy the physical appetite. They help transform food into the kind of brain chemistry that helps you move from the dining table to the sofa and then into the bedroom together.

It's not only the food you select, but the spices you use as seasoning. They can help swing the scales from "no" to "yes".

Who Says So?

The U.S. Department of Agriculture's Vitamin and Mineral Laboratory in Beltsville, Maryland. They issued a report on sluggish sugar metabolism which can produce a high insulin level in your body. The way you eat and how you season your food can bolster insulin's activity and help you regulate the blood sugar level in your body. This will provide more energy for daily activity and perhaps nighttime sex.

According to Richard A. Anderson, Ph.D., seasoning your diet with spices like cinnamon, clove, bay leaves, and some others can triple insulin's ability to control sugar. Somehow, the spices make insulin more efficient at removing sugar from the blood and converting it into useful energy.

High levels of insulin, produced by the body in response to sluggish glucose metabolism, are thought to promote illnesses such as atherosclerosis. By lowering circulating insulin levels, the spices discourage the formation of cholesterol-laden plaques on coronary artery walls. So, better heart and artery health should have a beneficial effect on sexual ability . . . and we're talking about spicing up your meals, not taking prescription drugs!

Healthy sexual appetites need other food parts as well, like vitamin E, zinc, unsaturated fatty acids, phenylalanine and phospholipids, to manufacture male and female hormones. These particulars are ignored in conventional cookbooks because sexual health is not usually a concern, and general health depends on a varied diet.

But we are not general people or sexual people, we are a blend of both, and catering to one facet of our being at the expense of the other doesn't make sense. A knowledge of love cookery is essential. It can help to foster harmony between the sexes by way of equal satisfaction.

The Queen of Sheba

The dark Queen of Sheba, was able to charm King Solomon into the bed chamber and their love tussles were so satisfying that trade treaties were made between the Hebrew nation and the land of Sheba.

It's said that a love brew prepared in secret by a special group of servants skilled in magic was the key to her stamina and the stallion-like stamina of her partners. Three times a day her servants prepared the potion for her and the king. Because it had to be prepared fresh, vegetables were gathered from the nearby fields three times a day as well.

Fortunately, one slave escaped from Sheba and founded a potion shop in what's now known as Great Britain where she achieved great success with the nobles. This is the formula she said she compounded for the Queen of Sheba:

Queen of Sheba's Super Sex Tonic

Take:

1/4 cup fresh cabbage juice
1/4 cup fresh carrot juice
1/4 cup fresh potato juice
1/2 teaspoonful crushed spearmint leaves
1/4 teaspoonful crushed cloves
1/8 teaspoonful Ceylon cinnamon

Mix furiously until all of the ingredients are completely blended.

Drink one cupful three times a day.

Once again, this is the formula that the escaped slave made public in a letter which was written during her lifetime but was not to be opened until after her death.

We don't know if these were all of the ingredients.

Was she still faithful to the queen and the promise she had made to keep her magic love mixture secret?

Will the use of this mixture turn you and your partner into the king and queen of sex?

Give it a shot . . . it can't hurt!

Vitamins and Sex

(See also Appendix, page 311)

From the foreplay to the bed, a good tussle burns up about 200 calories, the equivalent of a two-mile run. If you're particularly athletic, well-nourished, under little outside stress, you can burn up the calorie equivalent of the New York Marathon.

Each of us have the formidable task of putting from forty to fifty essential food factors into our body every day. Among them are vitamins (this chapter) and minerals (next chapter).

Because so many of our foods are highly processed before they reach the table and because so many nutrients are no longer present in their natural state, a good multi-vitamin/mineral formula, taken with your food, should be a part of your daily routine. Taken once or twice a day it can help to make up for the nutrients lost during processing.

Vitamin A

Besides being necessary for good vision and as a body protector, vitamin A is important for the health of your skin and the mucous membrane that coats the reproductive and sexual areas. Without vitamin A, membranes become dry and tend to itch and crack. Lubrication ceases and sex can become unpleasant. Vitamin A can be gotten from liver, eggs, yellow-orange fruit and dark-green vegetables. Butter and fish oil also contain vitamin A, as does any good vitamin supplement.

The B-Complex Vitamins

No one is really sure how many B-Complex vitamins there are. They are necessary for the burning of food for energy and for most other processes of every cell in your body.

Like most of the B-Complex, *pantothenic acid* is vital to hormone formation. We are prone to a deficiency of this vitamin because there is a higher tissue concentration than there is in most of the foods we eat.

A *vitamin B^6* (pyridoxine) deficiency can cause impotence in men. And, without it, the neurotransmitters norepinephrine and acetylcholine cannot be produced. If they are not available, sexual desire and ability are not available either.

Vitamin B^6 is involved in the conversion of food into energy. A lack of B^6 means the body can't use glucose for energy, and you try to have sex if you're too tired to turn over.

B^6 is found naturally in tuna, lentils, whole grains, rice, bananas, spinach, potatoes, cantaloupe and other fruits and vegetables. Liver, meat and poultry are also good sources and supply loads of energy besides.

Vitamin B^1 combines with phosphoric acid in the body to make a coenzyme form called thiamin pyrophosphate. This contributes to the manufacture of acetylcholine, the neurotransmitter which has so much to do with memory and sex.

This illustrates why cutting meat and eggs from the diet completely can contribute to fatigue. Fatigue will definitely cut into your happy bed time. Which should we be, longer lived, happy in bed, or a combination of both?

Vitamin B^2 deficiency can also affect your sex life by robbing you of energy since this vitamin is also involved in the body's energy-producing cycle.

Niacin, vitamin B^3, will alter your sex life by interfering with your nerves and your digestive system. On the other hand, it can enhance it by dilating the blood vessels leading to the sexual apparatus and stimulating circulation to the important extremities.

Choline is needed to make important brain chemicals and a lack of this material will defeat all chances for sexual activity.

Once more concerning B-Complex, a deficiency of vitamin B^{12} will cause the condition known as anemia and, with it, a powerful reduction in the desire for sex.

Vitamin C

Vitamin C affects the sex life directly through its role in iron metabolism, the formation of red blood cells, and the health of the adrenal glands. All these procedures influence your sex life.

Vitamin E

Vitamin E protects the hormones of the pituitary gland and the adrenals from destruction, and it also aids cellular respiration to increase available energy.

Essential Fatty Acids

Essential fatty acids are needed by the thyroid gland, the adrenals, the prostate gland and the cells which manufacture prostaglandins. (See also Appendix, page 295.)

So, maybe a balanced diet which includes all food types, even those deemed "unhealthy," plus a vitamin/mineral supplement can be the best aphrodisiac in the world.

Chinese Apple Salad

(Thanks to Gary Selden's *Aphrodisia*)

Core and thinly slice 2 large apples.

Blend a dressing made from the juice of one orange, 4 teaspoons of honey and a dash of brandy.

Garnish with raisins, walnuts and fresh cherries.

Honey is primarily levulose and dextrose plus tiny amounts of 13 other natural sweeteners. It also contains the vitamins and minerals needed by the body to digest its sugars. Honey contains one of the non-essential amino acids called *aspartic acid* which some doctors have used to treat "bedroom fatigue."

Don't be confused by the term non-essential. It is not that the amino acid is non-essential, it means that it can be manufactured in the body from the food you eat. Essential amino acids cannot be manufactured and must be obtained from food.

Minerals and Sex

(See also Appendix, page 297)

Vitamins get the press but minerals are even more important to your sex life.

Phosphorus

Phosphorus was the first mineral directly linked to sexual arousal. When phosphorus refiners, making matches in the days when wooden matches were the only ones available, got it on their hands every day, were perpetually erect and were forced to see their doctors, the link between this mineral and sex was discovered.

But don't run out and lick a match. The erection could continue until extremely painful, or worse, until gangrene set in.

Phosphorus is a deadly poison and it's much healthier to get it from organic sources like fish, eggs, milk, nuts, seeds and beans.

Need I mention once again that some of the phosphorus-containing foods are included in the no-no listing of some nutritional experts?

Zinc

Zinc is another sex mineral.

Both sexes make hormones with zinc but it's particularly important for sperm and seminal fluid. Zinc deficiency may be related to a loss of the sex drive. Try organ meats, oysters, eggs, raw nuts and seeds, whole grain cereals and caviar.

A lack of zinc may be responsible for sterility in some males and should be considered in all cases.

Zinc is concentrated in the pineal gland, the sex glands and the eyes, so be sure there is an adequate supply in your body.

Calcium

Calcium is great for bones but it also plays a big part in your sex life. Calcium affects the production of hormones by the endocrine glands, the menstrual cycle and the fertility of men and women.

Other effects of calcium on your sex life include steadiness of affection, strength in performance and the prevention of overexcitement. Glandular imbalance due to a deficiency can reduce sexual interest and ability.

Silicon

Silicon is never discussed because most people don't even know it exists. An enjoyable sex life is impossible without silicon. The outer covering of all the nerves in the body and the brain need silicon in order to be excited. Your hair, skin and nails are lifeless without silicon. This mineral makes you want to move and to live in joy and happiness.

If you need silicon you can get it in the health food store or drugstore. Food sources include rice polishings, sprouts, whole grains, and oat straw tea.

Sodium

Sodium from common salt. All body fluids, including sexual fluids, carry sodium salts so a little bit is necessary. You can get all you need from celery, veal or okra.

Potassium

Potassium affects human sexuality by insuring healthy nerve and muscle activity. Without sufficient potassium in your diet, you would be too weak to perform sexually even if the desire was there.

Sulfur

Sulfur helps keep the skin young and responsive and is a cleanser that keeps the sexual system free of impurities.

Magnesium

Magnesium is the relaxer. When your lifestyle keeps you too wound up to enjoy sex, magnesium relaxes you and enhances your enjoyment of the act.

Manganese

Manganese is needed in many enzyme reactions and is essential to human sexuality.

Selenium

Selenium is new on the essential mineral scene. It's routinely given to animals to ensure normal reproduction. Selenium-deficient rats are often sterile. While we know that selenium is important to our immune system, the effect on sexual activity is up in the air. Some men and women who have taken selenium in supplement form have stated that there was an increase in sexual desire, but there have not been studies done to prove this.

Vanadium

Vanadium deficiency slows the reproductive ability of rats but has not been tested in humans. Although little is known about this mineral, it appears to be important since it is present in every cell in the body. Main sources are corn, soy, olive oils and also black pepper.

Chocolate — Fact vs. Fiction

Chocolate will not give you acne.

Although peanuts and seafood can be troublesome to some allergy-prone people, few people are allergic to chocolate.

Chocolate will not cause headaches or worsen migraines. If you nibble on chocolate before a meal, the fat and sugar can kill your appetite.

Chocolate can evoke the pleasures of childhood, can be used as a means of easing disappointment and can help you get over a broken heart.

1.4 ounces in a chocolate bar does contain about 220 calories.

Chocolate alone won't cause cavities, but sugar and other fermentable carbohydrates *are* related to cavities. Chocolate contains no cholesterol, but the fat in cocoa butter is predominantly saturated. However, although most saturated fat tends to raise blood cholesterol, studies have shown that the fat in cocoa butter may be an exception. Studies in humans and animals have shown that cocoa butter has a neutral effect on blood cholesterol levels.

Chocolate contains phenylethylamine (PEA), an amphetamine-like chemical that helps to arouse emotions.

It's OK to treat yourself to chocolate on occasion, as part of an overall healthful diet, just don't overdo it.

Supplements You Never Heard of and Sex

Scientific studies have proved that individual foodstuffs have an effect on sexuality via their chemical constituents.

It's been shown that zinc is an important component of the male ejaculate. Casanova's purported habit of eating fifty oysters as his daily dinner may well have been one of the secrets of his success, for oysters are very rich in zinc.

Certain foods, such as ginseng and sarsaparilla, are known to stimulate the adrenal cortex, which is involved in the production of sexual hormones.

Carrots, yams, and pomegranate seeds have estrogen-related factors and can supplement deficiencies in women.

A lack of substances called histamines has been linked with an inability to reach orgasm in both men and women. The production of histamine has been linked to the presence of vitamins B^{6}, B^{12}, and folic acid.

If your "get up and go" went one day and never returned, a change of diet and some good vitamin pills can help you get back what you think you have lost forever. Of course, you may also need some other supplements to start your motor up.

Here's a few natural remedies to add to your regimen as additional insurance. They're available in health food and drugstores for the most part and are not too expensive. Give them a month or two to exert their influence.

B^{15}

Ever hear of vitamin B^{15}? No?

That's because it isn't a vitamin. It's a natural substance found in apricots.

Gary Seldin in his book, *Aphrodisia* (E.P. Dutton, 1979), writes that some users have reported an astounding surge of erotic interest as well as far more intense climaxes. Two rather surprising results from a substance first found in ordinary fruit.

Russian doctors claim that it raises energy by improving oxygen transport to the heart.

They also claim it aids protein synthesis and helps regulate steroid hormone levels in the body.

Chemically, B^{15} is N'-N dimethylglycine.

Muhammad Ali used B^{15} plus honey and vitamin B^{12} as a supplement to raise his strength when he fought for and regained the heavyweight title.

The Dallas Cowboys used it and so did the N.Y. Yankees.

But, the FDA doesn't want it to be sold in the U.S.! So why am I bothering to tell you about a substance you can't get?

B^{15} is dimethylglycine (DMG).

It's legal to buy trimethylglycine (TMG).

TMG breaks down in the body into DMG plus an extra methyl group for energy for sex and additional help against pollution.

Therefore, if your sexual malaise is due to fatigue, try some TMG along with some of the recipes in this book.

New Form of Vitamin B^{15}

B-vitamins are vital to the metabolism of fats and proteins and necessary for the maintenance of muscle tone. They're also important to prevent anemia. And now there's a new form of vitamin B^{15} that may be important to your love life. It's called dibencozide and you'll find it in health food stores.

It's a form of vitamin B^{15} that's more easily absorbed for muscle strength and tone. Weightlifters are using this new form to train better and longer, you can use it to make love better and longer.

Octacosanol

Dr. Carlton Fredericks, the dean of nutritional research, explained that although vitamin E in wheat germ has been given the credit for its stimulating qualities, it is really the octacosanol it contains that does the job.

Octacosanol does step up semen production in men and works to increase energy. It can relax muscles, step up a feeling of well-being, increase reaction time and other mechanisms involved in the sex game.

If the man in the family tends to nod off after dinner when you want to make love, this may be the answer.

Wheat germ makes a wonderful power food, but if it is not for you, octacosanol can be found in health food stores.

L-Phenylalanine

Here is an amino acid you can get in supplement form that will help make you or your mate more sexually aggressive. Stress and overwork can deplete most of the noradrenaline in your gray matter. It's the neurotransmitter in the brain that makes you want sex instead of sleep!

It's found naturally in eggs, meat and cheese but then it has to compete with other substances in trying to get into the brain area so it can be used. The better way is to use an amino acid supplement. Unless you have high blood pressure, PKU, or a pigmented melanoma, a small dose will serve to increase your sexual proclivities.

L-Tyrosine

L-Tyrosine is another amino acid which the body uses to prepare norepinephrine. It won't raise blood pressure the way that

L-phenylalanine will but it will help to raise anything else you have in mind.

Co-Enzyme Q-10

Co-Enzyme Q-10 is once again something new. It is essential for the production of energy in the body. It is considered to be in the ergogenic class (energy giver) and if you don't have enough in your body you won't have enough energy to turn this page.

Co-Enzyme Q-10 is part of the biochemical pathway from which adenosine triphosphate (ATP) and metabolic energy are derived to run individual cells and the entire body.

That's quite a job description. What it means is that this substance ferries fat into the cells to be burned for energy. That includes sexual energy. Your health food store has it on the shelf.

Gamma-Oryzanol

Gamma-oryzanol is a substance derived from rice bran oil. It is a work-enhancing, energy-producing substance that can effectively improve performance.

It appears that GO may also be able to increase the production of testosterone in the male. That means more sexy feelings and the ability to carry them out. Weightlifters are using this product to make them more capable of sustaining a workout.

It can do the same to your workouts as well.

Try your health food store or pharmacy.

L-Carnitine

L-carnitine is another member of the supplement staff that can be of benefit to your prowess.

It works in your body the way the carburetor in a car regulates the flow of gasoline. The flow determines how much fuel is burned to produce the power that keeps the wheels turning.

L-carnitine helps to regulate the rate at which your body burns fat for energy. The more there is present in your body, the more fat your body can burn and the more energy you have for any purpose you care to put it to.

Major sources of L-carnitine are meat and dairy products. If your doctor has advised that you must cut down on them for whatever good reason, you can find L-carnitine in the health food store along with the other supplements mentioned in this chapter.

Chromium

According to the USDA, only one person in ten gets even the minimum recommended amount of chromium (50 micrograms) in typical U.S. diets. The National Academy of Sciences recommends 50 to 200 micrograms daily.

It has been well-established that both exercise of any sort and sugar consumption increase the body's need for this mineral.

The shortage of chromium in so many diets creates serious problems which relate to energy and stamina. Insulin is an extremely important hormone. Minute by minute, it regulates the metabolism of carbohydrates, fats, and protein. These are the three major food categories necessary for your body to produce energy and to function. Biologically active chromium is absolutely essential if insulin is to do its job.

Body energy comes from burning blood sugar for the most part. The remainder comes from burning fats and protein. Insulin and chromium not only insure a rapid uptake of blood sugar but also assure its rapid conversion into glycogen — a special form of glucose which is stored for future energy needs and released as needed.

GTF chromium and chromium picolinate are two forms of chromium that can be purchased in health food stores and in drugstores in supplement form.

Arabian Nights

Here is the story of Ala-al Din abu-al and the pharmacist who prepared a love potion for him.

Touched by his story of a lack of amatory inclination, the pharmacist mixed equal parts of Chinese cubebs, cinnamon, cloves, cardamom, ginger, white pepper, and mountain shiek (a lizard), pounding them all together and boiling the mixture in olive oil, then adding a cupful of coriander seed and honey.

Take a spoonful of this mixture washed down with a sherbet made of rose conserve after eating a dish of lamb plentifully seasoned and hotly spiced.

(NOTE: There's enough fire in this potion to set off a volcano even if you leave out the lizard . . .)

Spices, Etc.

Sometime between the years 1394 and 1433, the manual of erotic techniques called *"The Perfumed Garden,"* was compiled by Sheikh al-Imam Abu Abd-Allah al-Nefwazi. It was translated into French and then into English by Sir Richard Burton.

There are twenty-one chapters dealing with coital techniques which you can investigate at your leisure and, although a good percentage of his writings prove him to be a wise man, some of his arguments are not always accurate. We shall restrict ourselves to the area dealing with aphrodisiac foods, even though some of his recipes are ridiculous.

Modern physicians would agree with many of his points about sound bodily health being of prime importance, while modern herbalists would agree with his contention that herbs and spices can contribute greatly to sexual health.

Two examples of fact and fancy:

"If you want to acquire strength for coitus, take the fruit of the mastic tree (derou, which is very nutritious) and pound it well with oil and honey. Drink of this liquid first thing in the morning; you will become vigorous . . . "

"The same result will be obtained by rubbing the virile member . . . with gall from the jackal. This rubbing stimulates those parts and increases their vigor."

Onion seed, cubeb pepper, ginger, cinnamon, cardamom, vinegar, garlic, nutmeg, long pepper, cloves and other spices are found in abundance in many of the "erotic formulas" designed to stimulate love or help increase both the quality and the quantity of amorous excursions.

Hot, spicy cooking has been introduced to the American table from Mexico, China, Morocco, the bazaars of India and the Far

East. The warm, musky aroma of dried spices has to increase your appreciation of the old sheikh's concept that spices are a prelude to lovemaking.

Did you think that Tex-Mex food was enjoyable just because the green chilies bit you on the way in?

What's more important to you is what they do on their journey to the way out!

Beans, chilies and onions, sometimes mashed with scallions for greater effect, plus some added peppers and cumin, tossed with vinegar and oil . . . wow!

The Cuban-Chinese cuisine is something else: Black bean soup laced with rum, fried rice, Chinese vegetables mixed with selected spices, fried plantains with chopped beef and olives — raisins — tomatoes — peppers! Again, wow!

Hungarians contributed the fantastic combination of meat, onions, fat, and pure ground paprika. Hot going down and stimulating for hours afterwards.

And we haven't considered Creole (French, Spanish, African, and Choctaw): Tomatoes, green pepper, onions, garlic, cayenne, Tabasco, sassafras and thyme!

What are these spices and how can you use them in your "Lover's Cooking?"

Allspice

This is not a mixture of many spices but the berry of the allspice tree which grows in the West Indies. Botanically it is called *Pimenta oficinalis* with common names of pimento, Clove pepper and Jamaica pepper.

It got the name Allspice because, when freshly ground, it tastes like a mixture of cinnamon, cloves and nutmeg. Use it in curries and Mexican dishes, and with beef, lamb, and chicken.

Anise

Botanically, *Pimpinella anisum,* it is an annual plant that has been used as an antispasmodic and aromatic carminative for centuries. The leaves are long and feathery and the seeds have the characteristic taste we associate with licorice.

Use anise in curries, stews, fish dishes, and with most cheese dishes . . . in moderation.

Cardamom

This is the dried fruit of a plant belonging to the ginger family, botanically known as *Elettaria cardamomum.*

The use of this spice began in India and it is one of the chief ingredients in curry powders. It has a strong flavor and has been suggested as a means of overcoming bad breath.

Cardamom is invaluable when making Indian dishes. It enhances the appeal of fish, chicken and even fruit compote. As an added kicker, try a drop in strong black coffee.

Cayenne

Capsicum frutescens, chili pepper and a host of other peppery names for this "hot" spice. It has been used as a general stimulant and to build up resistance at the first sign of a cold. It helps the digestion and, in small amounts, is excellent with eggs, cheese and shellfish. Tabasco sauce contains this spice.

Cinnamon

Cinnamomum zeylanicum. This is a bark usually sold in powdered form. It is stimulating to body organs. It is frequently used on appetizers such as cranberry sauce, spiced fruits, pickles and catsup. Whole pieces of the bark can be used with chutney. It can be sprinkled over ham, lamb, pork chops, beef stew, and as part of goose stuffing.

This pleasant smelling, versatile spice is also tossed over milk drinks, custard, baked apples and peaches. Try it in hot wine, tea, coffee or chocolate.

Cloves

Caryophyllus aromaticum. Cloves have been in use as long as mankind found that meat was good to eat. The unripened bud with its powerful odor was used to mask the smell of decaying meat before refrigeration. Many people dislike this herb because the smell reminds them of a dentist's office. The oil of clove is used as a local anaesthetic and will kill pain when placed in a cavity.

Cloves will also sweeten the breath and help digestion. They increase the flow of digestive juices permitting all of the nutrients to be extracted.

Excellent for sprinkling over baked fish, scrambled eggs, beets, sweet potatoes, tomatoes, spice cakes, cookies and puddings. Whole cloves are used in the marinade for beef, pork, lamb or veal.

Coriander

Coriandrum sativum. This is an herbal spice which has been considered to have aphrodisiac powers by directly stimulating the genital area.

It is used in many Mexican, Indian and Indonesian dishes. It is a basic to curry powder and is best when freshly ground. Try it in baking as well as when cooking sausage.

Cumin

Cuminum cyminum. The seeds are used in flavoring meat, cheese, eggs, hamburger, rice and other pilaff dishes. It looks and tastes a lot like caraway but is a little lighter. It is used in curry powders and in chili powders in Mexican, Indian, and North African cooking. Try it when baking bread or rolls. The taste and odor are stimulating.

Ginger

Zingiber officinale. Ginger is a root widely used in Chinese, Indian, African, Mexican and Southeast Asian cooking. When it is dried, it is more pungent than when cut from the raw root.

Chilies

Red and green chilies are used in the native cuisines of Mexico, Malaysia, Thailand, India, Pakistan, Africa and China. You can use them to enhance your sex life but you have to know how to use them because they're really hot!

To prepare fresh chilies, run them under cold water, cut off their tops and remove the seeds and veins. They can be peeled and scraped after charring over a gas flame, then wrapped in a towel. This makes them soft for cooking in sauces and enhances their flavor.

Dried chilies must be torn into small pieces and soaked in boiling water for 30 minutes before using. Use one cup of water to six chilies. This applies to dried chilies that are not to be powdered but put instead into a blender and puréed.

Chili powder is a blend of ground seeds and pods from dried chilies, mixed with other herbs and spices. You can buy a good chili powder but try to get it fresh because it loses potency after a year. One tablespoon of powdered chili equals one whole chili.

Some chili can sting your mouth or eyes so keep your hands away from your face when working with chilies or chili powder.

Mace and Nutmeg

Mace is the outer coating of the seed which grows on nutmeg trees in Sri Lanka, Sumatra, and Malaysia. Botanically named *Myristca fragrans*, the kernel yields the spice nutmeg. In small amounts, nutmeg is a stimulant but in large doses, it can be a hallucinogen and in larger doses can even be deadly.

Mace is milder and very fragrant and can be a substitute for nutmeg. Nutmeg is best when freshly grated but powdered nutmeg is more available in stores. Mace is especially tasty on trout, lamb and sausage. Try it on vegetables and potatoes. Also in puddings and on cottage cheese.

Nutmeg in Swedish meatballs, meat loaf and meat pie makes them a different meal. Also excellent in sauces over chicken, seafood and veal. And, of course, sprinkled on egg nog.

Fenugreek

This is the tiny reddish-brown seed from *Trigonella foenumgraecum*. It has a delightfully bitter flavor with a sweet and spicy scent when it is heated. It imparts part of the characteristic flavor to curry powder and is featured in many Indian dishes.

This herb has been considered an aphrodisiac by many people in the past and it still has that reputation today. It is one of the oldest medicinal plants and its use to help restore individuals to health after a severe illness dates back to the ancient Egyptians and to Hippocrates.

Horseradish

The piquant, biting taste of this root gives mustard its characteristic flavor. This herb should be used fresh if you prepare your own because it can become bitter if long-standing. Its sharp flavor is a wonderful foil to bland meats.

Mustard

Mustard grows in Asia, North Africa and Europe and is the spice most familiar to Americans. The seeds can be dark red or yellow. The dark seed is stronger than the light seed, but they are both used in sauces, pickles and curry powder. Ground mustard seed is especially good with sage when rubbed on pork roast.

Commercial dry mustard is a blend of both seeds, with a bit of turmeric to heighten the yellow. Prepared mustard is paste made with vinegar or wine, sugar and herbs.

Mustard often reflects the national temperament. French mustard is mixed with white wine, German mustard, with tarragon vinegar and spices; English mustard — like Chinese mustard — is a paste prepared from plain mustard powder and water.

Paprika

Columbus found paprika in the Caribbean Islands and brought it back to Europe. It comes from a species of capsicum plant, *Capsicum frutescens*, which is now cultivated in Central America, Europe, and the U.S.

Hungarian paprika is the most renowned; it is the strongest and is made from the whole pod, seeds, and stems of the dried red pepper. A milder Spanish variety is more commonly used in the United States, but look for the Hungarian paprika.

Paprika is rich in vitamin C (1 tablespoon is said to equal the juice of four lemons). It gives a sweet flavor to many dishes, including ground beef and all cheese mixtures. It is frequently used with chicken, pork chops and veal. It is a pleasant addition to a baked potato and adds flavor to salad dressings and cream sauces.

Recent research has found that, in addition to vitamin C, paprika contains large amounts of beta-carotene and vitamin A, B^1, B^2 and important minerals. Paprika stimulates the appetite, increases the flow of gastric juices, and has been used in the treatment of bronchitis, pleurisy, and joint afflictions.

Pepper

Black pepper is usually confused with the peppers of the capsicum family, but it is a berry that grows mainly in India, Southeast Asia, and the East Indies.

Its importance in overcoming the taste of rancid meat in the Middle Ages was reflected in its value. It was considered a source of wealth and was used to pay taxes. At the time of Henry II, its value was as great as silver and gold.

Pepper comes in several forms: powdered, coarsly ground, and as whole peppercorns. White pepper is merely pepper with the outer coating of the seed removed. It was an aesthetic inspiration designed to please people who dislike seeing black flecks in their food.

Saffron

Saffron is the dried stigma of an autumn crocus, native to Asia and parts of Europe. It is the most expensive spice in the world. A pound of saffron would require over 200,000 separate stigmata. It is sold as a powder or in tiny orange and gold threads. Unscrupulous packagers will adulterate the powder with the much cheaper herb turmeric so buy the threads when you can. They are usually sold in an envelope or in a vial.

Saffron is one of the earliest known spices and was popular with the Greeks, Babylonians, and Indians. In medieval Europe it was also used as a hair dye, and in Tibet monks use it to dye their robes.

This golden spice is used in Indian and Asian cooking and saffron rice is very popular. Stews and curries owe their color to the use of tiny amounts of saffron.

Saffron is still considered to be an aphrodisiac but beware . . . large doses can have a severe or even deadly effect! It contains an ingredient which can affect the central nervous system and damage the kidneys. Ten to twelve grams of saffron can be a fatal dose to a human. But, because it is so very expensive it is seldom used as a poison.

Follow cooking instructions, which usually call for one or two stigma, and you'll enjoy the flavor and effect with complete safety.

Turmeric

Turmeric is an Asian herb and is the dried aromatic root or rhizome of a plant related to the ginger family. Many Moroccan dishes owe their color to the use of turmeric curry.

Beverages

The Devil's Cup

In a large chafing dish, place two tablespoons of honey, two broken cinnamon sticks, six whole cloves, and the peel from half an orange and half a lemon. Add 1/2 cup of brandy.

Heat and stir.

When hot, ignite the brandy.

When the flame dies down, add four cups of freshly made strong coffee.

Ladle into demitasse cups and enjoy.

Coffee Viennese

Prepare a strong cup of coffee.

Add 1/8 teaspoon of ground cinnamon.

Add honey to taste.

Finish with a generous dollop of non-dairy whipped topping.

Cappuccino

Use tall, thin coffee mugs for this delight.

Pour in two-thirds hot espresso and one-third hot low-fat milk.

Sprinkle the top with ground cinnamon or ground nutmeg.

B&B Demitasse

To a demitasse cup of darkly roasted French coffee, add one ounce of B&B. Top with a dollop of non-dairy topping.

You can enjoy similar demitasses by using creme de menthe, anisette, or Galliano liqueur.

Coffee

Americans drink almost half of the world's supply of coffee. It started just after the Boston Tea Party removed the traditional cup of tea from American tables and has continued to this day.

The origin of coffee is misty and hidden in the veil of the Middle East. It is said that a group of monks were disturbed by the antics of a herd of goats grazing in a nearby field. Although goats usually sleep at sundown, these goats got friskier and more active as the hours passed. When some of the monks went out to the pasture, they found the goatherd out-frisking the goats.

After the goatherd confessed he had eaten of some red berries because his goats had enjoyed them, the monks reasoned that Mohammed had revealed a miracle to them, although in a dubious manner, which could keep them awake during their evening prayers. However the discovery was made, history records its entry as a popular drink when it was endorsed by the Mufti of Aden about 1454.

It may have been the Moslem answer to the ban on alcoholic beverages.

The Origin of Tea (Chinese Legend)

In the third millennium before the birth of Christ, Shen Nung, the emperor of China, was conceived as the result of a union between a princess and a dragon. Shen Nung was a great observer and he saw that those people in his vicinity who boiled their water before drinking suffered fewer diseases than those who drank directly from springs and wells.

Therefore, Shen Nung never drank unboiled water.

The wood which lit the fire which boiled the water was gathered by his servants from the trees which grew on his estate. They were wild camelia trees and tea trees.

One day, early in 2737 B.C., leaves from the tea tree fell into the boiling water. The emperor drank of the water and called it Ch'a. "It is", said the emperor, "a drink that gives vigor to the body, contentment to the mind and determination of purpose . . ."

Don't Think of Tea As Only a Cup of Tea

Tea Punch

2 quarts of iced tea
2 cups of pineapple juice
2 tablespoons lime juice
Spring of fresh mint
Honey to taste

Makes ten servings.

Party Punch

2 quarts iced tea
2 cans frozen lemonade
2 cans frozen limeade
2 cups cranberry juice
2 bottles of ginger ale

Serves a lot of people

Hot Spiced Tea

2 quarts of water
12 tea bags or 4 tablespoons loose tea
1/2 teaspoon whole cloves
1/2 stick cinnamon
1/4 cup lemon juice
1/2 cup orange juice
Honey to taste

Georgian Tea

6 tea bags
3 cups peach nectar
3 cups water
1 teaspoon whole cloves
Honey to taste

Bring nectar, water and cloves to a boil, simmer 5 minutes, pour over tea bags, cover and brew for 5 minutes. Remove tea bags and cloves. Add honey to taste.

The Origin of Tea (Indian Legend)

Perhaps the Chinese legend of the origin of tea is not satisfying to you. Try the Indian legend on for size.

There once was an Indian monk called Dharma who travelled to Nanking where he made a vow to sit in meditation before a wall for nine years without sleep. As time went by, Dharma began to feel drowsy and, after five years had passed, he actually dozed for a moment or two. Upon awakening, he was filled with remorse at his lack of faith and removed his eyelids which he threw to the ground. Immediately, a bush sprang up bearing delicate, shiny, tapered leaves. Upon chewing the leaves, the holy man was instantly refreshed, sleep was banished and he was able to resume his meditations for the rest of the allotted time.

Vermont Slurp

5 tea bags

2-3 tablespoons maple syrup

4 cups of water

1 teaspoon ground cinnamon

3/4 cup low-fat vanilla ice cream

Place the tea bags, syrup, cinnamon in a teapot, pour in 4 cups of boiling water, cover and let stand for 5 minutes.

Remove tea bags, pour into cups and then top with ice recream.

SEE, THERE'S MUCH MORE TO TEA THAN YOU IMAGINED!

Where Did Tea Bags Come From?

They were invented by a New York tea and coffee merchant who, in 1904, sent samples of tea, sewn by hand into silk bags, to his special customers. The answers he got were requests for more tea bags. His clients had discovered that it was much faster and easier to pour boiling water over the bag than to prepare a sample from loose tea. This unintentional bit of advertising resulted in the paper tea bag you use today.

Apple Tea

5 tea bags
4 cups apple juice
1 cup water
3 whole cloves
4 whole allspice
4 cinnamon sticks

Bring the apple juice, water, cloves, allspice and cinnamon sticks to a boil. Pour over the tea bags and let brew for five minutes.

Tea

Tea is a stimulating and satisfying drink to half the people in the world. The tea leaves are harvested, dried and crushed, then left to stand in cool fermentation sheds. Later, they are dried with bursts of hot air. It is then that the tea develops its aroma and black color. The best known of this type is orange pekoe.

Green tea, an unfermented type, is produced by drying the picked leaves, rolling them to break down the tannin-containing cells and redrying them.

Jasmine tea is produced by drying the tea leaves together with jasmine flowers. It has the flavor of green tea, the color of black tea and the aroma of jasmine.

Don't steep tea for too long a time because the tannin can interfere with the digestive process. Besides, it makes the tea bitter instead of delicious.

The stimulant in tea is called theine and is identical to the caffeine found in coffee and other beverages found in various countries.

Tea and Jam

5 tea bags
4 cups of water
1/2 cup apricot preserves

Place the tea bags and preserves in a teapot, pour in 4 cups of boiling water, cover and let brew for five minutes.

Remove tea bags and serve.

What Is There In Coffee, Tea And Cocoa That Is Stimulating?

We know about the caffeine which is a central nervous system stimulant. But there are also other closely related substances such as theophylline and theobromine to pep up activity. All are stimulating to brain function, cardiac action and gastric motion, and they can also act as diuretics (water pills).

Caffeine belongs to a group of compounds scientists call methylated xanthines, of which theophylline is also found in tea and theobromine in cocoa.

Coffee is the strongest of the three beverages. The caffeine content of coffee is two to three times that of tea or cola drinks (about 100 to 150 milligrams of caffeine per cup of coffee compared to 30 to 70 milligrams per cup of tea or 10 to 12 milligrams in the average 12 ounce cola drink.)

A cup of coffee can increase your alertness, make you think more clearly, increase your attention span, shorten your reaction time and even improve your sexual reaction as well.

Who Says?

According to Doctor Judith Wurtman, prominent nutrition researcher at Massachusetts Institute of Technology, caffeine can enhance athletic performance. Isn't sex play a type of athletic performance?

And What About Cocoa?

It was in 1502 that Columbus first tasted cacao in the land we know as Honduras. It was served in the traditional Mayan fashion — dark, unsweetened, ground and roasted, then mixed with corn beer. Columbus was not impressed. Evidently the Mayans were, since the beans were so esteemed that they served as money throughout the Mayan Yucatan. Linnaeus considered this tradition when he named the tree *Theobroma,* "food of the gods." Where did its reputation as a nutritious food and sexual stimulant come from?

It was a thousand miles down the coast and at a different time that Cortes and his retinue came upon cocoa again in the Aztec capital named Tenochtitlan. But this time was different. It was in the form of *xoxo-atl,* a delicious, mouth-appealing beverage sweetened with honey, flavored with *thilxochitl* (vanilla), and chilled by snow brought by runners from the mountains.

Café Chocolat

Combine equal parts of darkly roasted French or Italian coffee with hot chocolate.

Top with non-dairy whipped cream.

Sprinkle some ground cinnamon or grated orange peel on the fluffy topping.

Ecstasy!

Every day in the court of Montezuma, at least two thousand cups of cocoa were served, with Montezuma accounting for as many as fifty cups himself. Considering the number of women in his harem, this was just enough.

Cocoa is low in vitamins but rich in minerals which are not destroyed by the heat of processing. Like all beans, cocoa contains a fair amount of protein and is especially rich in phosphorus. Its combination of this mineral, theobromine and its unique taste is pleasurable to the mouth and stimulating to shared caresses.

Consider this delightful way to end the dinner and prelude a night's romance.

Beer, Wine and Sex

Beer can help you keep your body free from toxic elements.

This means your body can have more fun in bed because you have eliminated some of the environmental products which cause fatigue and depression.

Who says so?

Researchers at the University of Minnesota have found that hops, the ingredient in beer that makes the brew have that wonderfully bitter taste, contains ingredients that help your body eliminate toxins, poisons, pollutants, chemicals and other unwanted materials.

The ingredients in hops are called lupulones and humulones. They stimulate your liver to make extra quantities of enzymes which are able to digest and get rid of harmful substances. So, a beer with dinner can be a sex aid, but only one beer!

One glass of wine can also remove inhibitions, make you and your partner feel free . . . but only one glass 'cause two or more can defeat the sex act entirely.

Even More Stimulating And Restorative Beverages

The French Court had many interesting ways to revive a flagging ambition.

We are not interested in alcoholic intoxication, but in the release of inhibitions.

Pousse-L'Amour (Love's Liqueur)

Put into a Madeira glass:

1/4 glass Maraschino
The yoke of an egg
1/4 glass of Madeira
1/4 Creme de Cacao
1/4 glass Brandy

Vin Tonique Et Aperitif (Tonic and Appetizer Wine)

In two pints of white Bordeaux wine, steep

1/6 ounce of juniper berries
1/2 ounce of Peruvian Bark
1/2 ounce of Quassia chips

Let stand for ten days.

Filter the liquid and add an equal amount of syrup of orange peel.

Drink one glass a day as a restorative.

Vin Aphrodisiaque (Wine d'Amour)

Take two pints of a good Chablis
Mix in one ounce of vanilla
One ounce cinnamon bark
One ounce ginseng
One ounce grated rhubarb.

Let stand for 15 days, stirring every day.

Filter and have a drink every day.

Aphrodisiaque Abyssin

While we do not recommend sugar, this mixture will not lend itself to the use of honey.

Prepare in a Pyrex-type glass:

Two lumps of sugar
4 drops of Curacao
1 glass of red Port wine (small glass)

Fill the glass with water and then warm almost to a boil.

Serve with a slice of lemon and grated nutmeg.

Recipes from the Renaissance

A good cook did not refer to written instructions about amounts. He or she cooked with a "pinch" of this and "so much" of that. These recipes are written for the cook who wants to control the kitchen.

Egg Yolks & Wine

Beat six egg yolks and slowly add a glass of Madeira.

Then, little by little, blend in a cup of cold chicken broth and a teaspoonful of powdered cinnamon.

Pass through a sieve.

Cook in an earthenware pot over low heat after adding a bit of butter.

When it thickens, pour it into cups.

Serve hot with nutmeg and a sprinkle of sugar.

Eggs and Anchovies

Cut equal amounts of some shallots, black olives and fillets of anchovies into small pieces.

Fry lightly in Canola oil or Olive oil.

Add three finely sliced Spanish peppers (pimiento).

Beat the eggs and mix with the above ingredients.

Put a spoonful of oil in a frying pan and add the mixture when the oil is hot.

Cook as you would an ordinary omelette.

Serve with crusty bread and with or without tomato sauce.

Breast of Chicken with Truffles

Prepare some chicken breasts by removing the skin and washing well. Rub them with red and black pepper and a bit of salt.

Line a heavy frying pan with thin slices of ham.

Put the breasts on top, sprinkle them with chopped parsley, crushed basil and a few seeds of fennel.

Fry until well colored.

Take an oven-proof dish and transfer the food to it. Place on top a thick layer of sliced truffles and a glass of good sherry.

Put into a 350° oven for a few minutes or until the wine bubbles and the aroma is exciting.

Remove and serve.

Snails à la Keats

Buy fresh snails and put them in an earthenware bowl with a lid.

For two weeks feed them milk. This is done by pouring a glass of milk over the snails every morning.

When cooking time arrives, put the snails into another dish and add to cover a mixture of water, vinegar and salt. Leave them covered in the infusion overnight.

In the morning, wash them well under the tap and place them in boiling water.

After this, remove them from their shells, dip them in beaten eggs and fry them in olive oil. Before serving, dip them into a sauce made from fish stock, coriander, rue, and lovage.

Delicious!

Almond Soup

Take a quart of fresh almonds and blanch them.

Put them in a mortar and grind them finely.

Add the yolks of six eggs and grind to a fine paste.

Mix slowly, and in parts, with a quart of chicken stock.

Mix in a quart of low fat milk.

Stir well, place in a pot over medium heat.

Stir continuously until piping hot.

Serve.

Celery Cream Soup

Peel a bunch of celery, scald it and cut into small pieces.

Put the pieces in a pan with some butter, a sprinkle of flour, two cups of good chicken broth, the yolk of one egg, 2 ounces of low-fat milk and a dash of nutmeg.

Heat and serve piping hot.

Caviar and Eggs

Fish eggs and hen's eggs, mixed in this exotic dish, guaranteed the attention of the most exhausted male. If he didn't respond to this creation it was time to call in the priest!

Mix together:

Four fresh eggs, well beaten
A small spoonful of grated bread
Pinch of chopped chives
Pinch of parsley
A little grated lemon peel
2 teaspoons of caviar

Heat some butter in a frying pan and when hot add the mixture as if you were making a pancake.

When cooked on one side, turn it over and cook the other side.

Serve flat with some crunchy French bread.

Eggs Gruyère

Save your stale bread, but before it goes moldy try this egg dish:

> *Poach some eggs*
>
> *Put them on pieces of toast, sprinkle with a bit of cayenne pepper, then cover thickly with Gruyere cheese.*
>
> *Place them on a baking sheet and brown them in a hot oven.*

How Many Eggs?

Two for each of you.

Breakfast?

Not necessarily, unless you want to be late for work! It's better in the evening accompanied by a small glass of red wine.

The Eggsistential Egg

Three eggs a week can't hurt!

Eggs do contain cholesterol but they also contain enough lecithin to emulsify said cholesterol.

They also contain, on average, 7 grams of the highest quality protein, with the essential amino acids in the proper proportion, for you to use in building and repairing your body.

Eggs contain significant amounts of all vitamins except vitamin C. They are rich in vitamins A, E, B-Complex and D.

Eggs supply large amounts of calcium, iron, potassium and sexy phosphorus. Eggs also have sulfur.

Free range eggs may be better for you than the usual eggs found in the markets. Free range eggs come from chickens which have been allowed to run free and supplement their diet naturally with bugs, grass, seeds, worms, etc.

Try Madame DuBarry's Deviled Eggs

Hardboil a dozen eggs.

Cut them carefully in half lengthwise and remove the yolks.

Mix the yolks with some truffles and some paté de foie gras.

Stuff the egg halves with the mixture and place them in a casserole lined with Canadian bacon.

Add some Madeira, a pinch of salt, pepper and nutmeg.

Cover and poach in the oven.

Brains of Veal à la Mustafa

Scald two brains of veal in boiling water and clean well.

Put them up in white wine with a *bouquet garni* of one clove of garlic, a sprig of rosemary, two cloves, a few leaves of parsley and a small piece of celery.

Boil some white onions and add to the pot.

When the brains are cooked, remove the *bouquet garni*.

Slice some truffles over the brains and serve hot.

Fried Beef Brain

Scald the brain in hot water and clean well, then chop into ten pieces.

Mix together a little flour, chopped parsley, chopped chives, and a pinch of allspice.

Roll the pieces of brain in the mixture to allow the brains to be coated.

Heat some olive oil in a frying pan and fry gently until done.

Kidneys and Champagne

Take some kidneys and cut them into thin slices.

Put them into a saucepan with a bit of olive oil, a pinch of salt and pepper.

Add a pinch of nutmeg and sliced mushrooms.

When the kidneys are almost done, add a pinch of flour and a glass of champagne.

When the kidneys are done, remove them from the pan and serve with a squeeze of lemon over them.

Sweetbreads with Mushrooms

Parboil the sweetbreads and clean them well.

Cut them into small pieces and put them in a saucepan.

Add a little olive oil and a pinch of salt and pepper.

Sauté for five minutes.

Slice the mushrooms and truffles and add them to the pot with a cup of broth.

Let cook slowly over a moderate flame for ten minutes.

Serve.

Mushrooms Bordelaise

Take some large mushrooms.

Clean them, remove the stalks and make a small incision on the top.

Soak them in olive oil, pepper and a pinch of salt for about two hours.

Meanwhile, make a hash of garlic, parsley and thyme.

Take the mushrooms out of the marinade and put them on the grill.

Cover them with the hash and moisten them with the marinade as they grill.

Before serving, sprinkle them with a bit of lemon juice.

(You'll never consider mushrooms the same way again once you've tried this dish.)

Breast of Chicken with Truffles

Prepare some chicken breasts, season with a little salt and pepper.

Line a frying pan with thin slices of ham and put the breasts on top of the ham.

Sprinkle some parsley, basil and ground fennel over them.

Cook until done.

Arrange the breasts in an oven-proof dish and put a thick layer of truffles on top of them.

Add a glass of good sherry wine and heat in the oven for a few minutes.

Serve piping hot.

Casanova, Don Juan, Cleopatra, Henry VIII

Who hasn't heard of the sexploits of these legendary lovers.

Was it secret combinations of foods which enabled them to satisfy themselves and their lovers... again and again?

Suspend your disbelief and silence your inner critic for a moment to partake of some of the "explanations" of their enviable abilities. These stories that have been passed down to us are part fact and part fancy. Pick the "wheat" from the "chaff" and you too may become a legendary lecher in your own time...

Don Juan was a 14th-century aristocrat who was born in Seville, Spain. He had the startling ability to make love to one maiden after another, competing with much younger men, but able to continue long after they had withered, and this power remained with him till he was well past 70.

According to written reports which surfaced after his death, he credited a particular mixture with the power to restore his potency time after time. It had to be mixed fresh and taken one hour before his next encounter.

Don Juan's Secret Passion Potion

Take 1/4 teaspoon of crushed basil leaves and 1 cup of freshly squeezed tomato juice.

Mix furiously until the fragrance from the basil has entirely entered the juice.

Sip slowly until the potion works its way to the genital area.

Now this is the published version of Don Juan's fantastic love potion. It's possible that not all of the ingredients were revealed. The Don was a tricky fellow and was careful not to reveal the secret during his lifetime. Did he add some cinnamon, Chinese licorice or perhaps some ginseng? Or is this the entire potion, able to do for you what it did for the Don?

Courtesans' Concoctions

Although most stimulating dishes simply evolved out of folklore, we do know the origin of some famous recipes. We are aware of those culinary preparations which ensnared and dominated the mind and body of King Louis XV. He was tantalized and teased by the talents of Madame de Pompadour, Madame duBarry, and Madame de Maintenon.

Before him, Louis XIV ate Cotelettes à la Maintenon to revive a flagging ambition. Francis the First found the famous dish, Frangipane, prepared by Catherine de Medici, to be the answer to his amorous prayers.

So, without further convincing recourse to the validity of these recipes, we begin an exploration of those considered to be the most efficacious.

Cotelettes de Veau à la Maintenon

Veal Cutlets prepared in a special way

2 thick cutlets of lean veal
2 slices of ham
4 medium onions
1 small bunch of parsley
3 scallions
1/2 Laurel leaf
2 cloves
Pinch of sweet basil
Pinch of coriander
1 can of anchovies

In a casserole dish, wrap the cutlets with the ham slices and the anchovies. Chop the onions and scallions with the rest of the ingredients and add to the casserole.

Bake in the oven at 350° for ten minutes. Cover with a few spoonfuls of brandy and put back in the oven for an additional ten minutes.

Serve over cooked brown rice using the gravy to moisten both the cutlets and the rice. Goes very well with one glass of red wine.

Frangipane

Almond cake

This innovative almond cake stirred kings and princes to amorous excesses. Here is the recipe, see what you can do with it!

2 oz heavy cream
3 egg whites
1 teaspoon vanilla
1 oz sugar
1 oz honey
1 cup of almond paste

Preheat oven to 300°F. Mix almond paste with sugar and honey, mold with fingers until blended. Add egg whites, cream and vanilla. Blend into a soft dough that will hold its shape when dropped from a spoon. Spoon onto an oiled cookie sheet. Bake twenty minutes — then go to it!

Fillets de Soles à la Pompadour

2 fillets of sole washed and paper-towelled to dry.
6 large mushrooms, chopped
1 oz Bordeux wine
1 oz cider vinegar
1 teaspoon ground ginger
1 tablespoon canola oil
2 tablespoons soy sauce
1 egg yolk

In a skillet, heat oil and add vinegar and wine, add fillets and cook until fish flakes. Sprinkle mushrooms over the tops of fillets, moisten with soy sauce and sprinkle with ginger. Take a tablespoon of sauce and mix with egg yolk, return to pan and sauté for three minutes. Turn fillets and cook 3 minutes.

These extravagant menus are culled from the annals of French history and bear the name of the historical character that used and swore by their efficacy. Le Compte De Mirabeau was an orator and revolutionary leader (1749-1800). Maybe the following dish can revolutionize your love life.

Cailles à la Mirabeau

2 stalks of celery
1 cup of sherry wine
2 quail
1/2 cup of raisins
2 tablespoons canola oil
1 carrot, slivered
1 onion, diced
3 mushrooms or truffles, sliced
2 tablespoons butter

Preheat oven to 450°F, wash and dry the quail, sprinkle inside and out with salt and pepper. In a casserole pour wine and butter (melted) and canola oil. Baste quail in mixture and bake for five minutes. Add chopped celery, the slivered carrot and diced onion, sprinkle raisins over quail and vegetables. Reduce the heat to 350° and roast for twenty minutes. Baste and add mushrooms. Bake for ten minutes more. Serve hot as a one dish meal. Vive l'amour!

Tendrons d'Agneau au Soleil

(Tendrons or medallions of lamb for Sun Kings)

The colors and textures in this dish, as well as the aroma, stimulate erotic desire. Try this dish served on a red table cloth with candles and a rose or two floating in a brass bowl.

4 lamb medallions
1 cup of beef broth
6 white mushrooms
Minced shallots, parsley, lemon pepper, garlic salt
1 slice of bacon
1/2 cup red wine
1/2 cup red vinegar

Marinate the medallions in a mixture of red wine, wine vinegar, parsley, lemon pepper, garlic salt for 1 or 2 hours in the refrigerator.

In a saucepan, melt the bacon slice for a few minutes, then add sliced mushrooms. Sauté for ten minutes, add beef broth, add marinated medallions and herbs. Simmer for thirty minutes, uncovered, stirring occasionally.

Serve hot with a small dish of cherry preserves (optional).

DuBarry was expert in the art of seduction. She secured her place in the heart of Louis XV through her knowledge of the pleasures of love. She kept her royal lover in a state of addiction and intoxication. Many of the mysterious secrets she used pertained to arousing cookery. She learned some of her tricks, in the bedroom and out, from a friar named Lange when she was placed in a convent upon her arrival in Paris. From there she moved into the home of a fashionable dressmaker, sieur Labille, and then became a companion to Dame de la Verrière. It was there she was introduced into the art of love in earnest.

The following recipes come from her collection of culinary marvels that are said to have kept her lover in a state of frenetic sensualism.

Les Ris de Veau à la Ayen

Sweetbreads à la Ayen

2 sweetbreads
1/2 pimiento
1 garlic, chopped
3 shallots, chopped
3 sprigs parsley, chopped
1 oz mixed nuts
1 tablespoon flour
1/2 cup dry white wine
1/2 cup beef stock
1/2 cup chicken stock
3 tablespoons butter
1 egg yolk stirred into 2 tablespoons milk

Soak sweetbreads in ice water for one hour. Drain and put into boiling water to cover. Simmer ten minutes. Preheat oven to 350°. In a flameproof casserole, melt the butter, then add the shallots, pimiento (slivered), parsley, and garlic. Cook slowly until the shallots are golden. Add trimmed sweetbreads, wine, beef stock, chicken stock, egg and milk mixture and a dash of pepper. Dust with flour and bake for thirty minutes. Grind the nuts and sprinkle over the dish.

Serve hot and tempting.

DuBarry culled many culinary techniques from mentors, one of them was the dressmaker/courtesan Labille whose specialty was dominance.

Her lovers were subdued with an appeal to all their senses. She would set a scene using colors and scents, soft pillows and other enticements. Then, through food, she plunged them into a delight of aromas, textures, taste combinations, and profusions of verbal reinforcements. The dishes were reputedly aphrodisiac. The following is one of her recipes.

Labilles' Les Fillets de Sole à la Soubise

2 fillets of sole
1/2 cup port wine
3 or 4 diced mushrooms
6 asparagus tips, 2 cloves of garlic, a pinch of thyme, puréed
3 tablespoons butter
2 tablespoons heavy cream

Sprinkle fillets with salt and pepper and simmer or poach in water to cover for about 8 minutes. Add wine, butter, heavy cream and mushrooms, bring to a boil. Add the puréed asparagus, garlic and thyme. Let boil for one minute, let set for one minute. Remove to platter and garnish with leaves of mint and thin slices of golden pepper (optional, choose your own garnish). Serve hot.

After Labilles' instructions, duBarry studied with the famous procuress at GOURDAN, where she learned how to accentuate desire with food. One of her favorite recipes was:

Les Oeufs de Poulet

Love letters à la duBarry. (Poulet means love letter or chicken)

4 hardboiled eggs
1/2 cup Madeira wine
2 tablespoons flour dissolved in beef broth
Bouquet garni (of herbs)
Rasher of bacon
2 tablespoons beef gravy
Salt, pepper and a dash of nutmeg
2 artichoke hearts (vinaigretted or cooked)

In a fireproof casserole, place bacon. Sprinkle with salt, pepper and nutmeg. Place over hot stovetop flame until bacon is melted. Remove and add artichoke hearts, flour in beef broth, wine and bouquet garni. Add beef gravy and place eggs in a row down the center. Place dots of gruyère (optional) and bake for thirty minutes at 350° in oven. Remove and serve hot.

Other Dainties Served by duBarry

Ginger Omelet

Dissolve four ounces of flour in a glass of low-fat milk.

Put through a sieve into a casserole dish.

Into that mixture, add 1/2 teaspoon of butter and two teaspoons of powdered sugar and stir over gentle heat until thickened.

Take off the flame and stir until firm.

Warm the mixture once again, then take it off the flame, add four ounces of pulverized ginger and six egg yolks, beaten.

Whip the egg whites and add them to the mixture, stirring.

Then, pour everything into the casserole and place it in a slow oven.

When the mixture is puffed up to a golden brown dome, remove from the heat, sprinkle with just a whitening of powdered sugar and serve.

(This is not a diet dish, nor is it for the cholesterol-conscious individual, but once in a while it can work miracles.)

Oysters duBarry

Get two dozen oysters, wash them well and drain. Put them back in their shell and bake for five minutes.

Meanwhile:

Take a bunch of spinach
2 onions
A bunch of parsley
Head of lettuce
2 tablespoons Worcestershire sauce
3 tablespoons anchovy sauce
1 ounce of Parmesan cheese
Sprinkle of salt
3 drops Tabasco sauce

Genitalia

It should come as no surprise that animal parts other than muscle meat and organ meat have been given a role in sexual restoration.

Gonadotropic concentrates, residing in the private parts of animals have been credited with the ability to inspire a diminished libido.

Even the indefatigable Madame de Pompadour, when tired from love's tussles, ate prepared testicles. It appeared that the testosterone stimulation made her more womanly.

The simplest way to prepare them is to remove the outer membrane and sauté them in olive oil, cooking slowly on all sides.

Cartolomeo Scappi, private chef to Pope Pius V, prepared bull's balls pie using this recipe:

Boil 4 bull's testicles in 2 cups of chicken broth.

Remove the outer membrane when tender and slice finely. Sprinkle them with cinnamon, nutmeg, white pepper and a pinch of salt.

Cook a mincemeat of 1 pound lamb's kidneys, 1/4 pound lean ham, 4 cloves garlic, 1/2 teaspoon each of thyme and marjoram.

Line a pie plate with pastry, then cover the bottom with ham. Add a layer of testicle, then one of mincemeat and continue until the pie is filled. Add a glass of wine before adding the top crust.

Bake at 400 degrees for about fifteen minutes or until the crust is done and the filling has cooked through.

(NOTE: Please, no letters. I do not know why the Pope's chef prepared this dish. Maybe it was for visiting dignitaries outside of the church.)

Chop the greens finely. Mix with breadcrumbs softened with butter and the rest of the ingredients, except the cheese. Pour the sauce over the oysters, top with finely minced breadcrumbs and grated Parmesan cheese and bake until brown.

Serve hot.

Louis XV was a pretty good cook himself. He made this dish for himself and his mistresses:

Macaroon Omelet

Take the yolks of six eggs and six ounces of powdered sugar, mix vigorously.

Beat the whites separately and when they are fluffy as snow, mix with the yellows.

Pound six macaroons until very fine and add to the mix.

Heat some butter in a frying pan and when hot, pour in the omelet.

Cook slowly until done, then serve.

He also made a pretty good brains and oysters soup:

Brains and Oysters Soup

First boil the brains, clean them and let cool until they can be handled.

Cut into pieces and mix them with a combination of eggs and bread crumbs previously fried in olive oil.

Using the same olive oil, add some flour (tablespoonful), chopped parsley, black pepper and a handful of oysters and broth.

Heat everything together and serve with French bread on the side.

Products From The Sea

As a source of sexual-stimulating phosphorus, zinc and other minerals important to sexual health, products from the sea have to be considered the best.

The similarity between blood and seawater with traces of magnesium, sodium, chloride, potassium, calcium and sulfates supports our beginnings. Even fatty fish has less calories than fatty meats and less fat. Levels of amino acids are about the same for sea animals as land animals. Oysters, the food that folklore suggests as the best support for the ailing male, has ten times more zinc per weight than any other food!

Alexander the Great was told about sturgeon roe by Darius. Alex was called great . . . not because of all of the lands he conquered. The Roman emperors would have teams of runners deliver fresh fish in tubs of sea water from the Caspian Sea.

Ah! caviar . . . 100 grams of which contain 355 milligrams of bioactive phosphorus, 276 milligrams of calcium, a smattering of assorted vitamins, enzymes and 27 grams of protein.

Frog's Legs à la Bordelaise

Fry the frogs legs, seasoned with a pinch of salt and pepper, in a shallow pan in very hot, but not smoking, olive oil.

When golden-brown on both sides, place them on a plate with a squeeze of lemon juice and a pinch of parsley.

Caviar Canapé

Toast some rounds of bread.

Butter lightly.

Take some hardboiled eggs and slice them.

Press the whites of the egg on the rounds of bread to make a circle.

Inside of the circle, place the caviar.

Over the top sprinkle some minced onion and minced egg yolk.

This dish looks pretty, tastes wonderful and is a potent stimulant to the libido.

Caviar and Anchovy Canapés

Cut some rounds of bread and sauté lightly in olive oil.

Spread these with caviar.

Top with minced egg yolk.

Place a stuffed olive in the center.

Arrange on a plate with fillets of anchovy.

Potage d' Haricots

Soups and purées should be served very hot and especially the bean soups and bean purées. Use any large bean: red kidney, fava, chick peas or lima beans. If you do not want to cook them, the canned variety is satisfactory but make sure you drain them thoroughly. Use a 16 oz can or the cooked equivalent.

Use one quart chicken stock, or four packets of chicken broth in one quart of water. Add a pinch of saffron and a handful of finely chopped parsley. Bring to a boil and add the beans until well cooked. Place in a food processor and purée. Save a few whole beans for garnish. Heat and serve with whole bean garnish and grated parmesan cheese. Serves two.

Consommé Vivier

Take a strong consommé, homemade or canned, about 1 quart. Bring to a lively boil. In a food processor, purée celery, tomato, basil, thyme and rosemary. Use a few spoons of consommé for consistency. Return to saucepan. Cook uncovered for five minutes. Sprinkle with parsley garnish, add a few spoonfuls of sweet cream and serve at once. An added garnish of chopped chervil is optional. Serves two.

Caviar Omelette

4 eggs, well beaten
2 tablespoons bread crumbs
A pinch of chopped chives and parsley mixed with caviar of choice
1 teaspoon lemon peel, grated

Place butter in a frying pan and melt until it bubbles, then place the mixture in so that it covers the bottom of the pan, as in making pancakes. Cook until ready to turn over, then do the other side. Serve hot for two.

Pimiento Omelette

4 eggs well beaten
Olives stuffed with pimiento, sliced, about 12
Pinch of Cayenne pepper
Spanish peppers, sliced

Place butter in frying pan and melt until it bubbles. Mix ingredients with eggs and make omelette in the usual way.

Easter Egg Rice

2 eggs beaten
3 cups of chicken broth
3/4 cup cooked rice
Grated parmesan cheese

Into a saucepan place the chicken broth and rice and bring to a boil. Mix the eggs and cheese and put into broth. Stir continuously until strands of egg solidify. Serve hot in deep bowls, garnish with grated nutmeg. Serves two.

Chestnut Soup

1 quart of chicken stock, or four packets of M.B.T. chicken broth in quart water
1 eight oz jar of peeled chestnuts
3 oz of lean smoked bacon
2 sprigs of fennel, plus one for garnish
8 oz of plain yogurt
Freshly ground black pepper to taste
Salt to taste

In a large saucepan, bring broth or chicken stock to boil over high heat. Add the chestnuts, bacon, fennel and salt and pepper. Simmer over medium heat for 40 minutes. Remove saucepan from heat, discard the bacon. Using a slotted spoon, remove the chestnuts from the broth and place in a food processor. Add two teaspoons of broth and process to a purée. Pour the purée back into the pan, add the yogurt and stir well. Heat gently and serve garnished with fresh sprig. Yield: two servings.

Seafood, Your Thyroid Gland and Feeling Sexy

Your thyroid gland controls the rate at which your body produces energy to cook, drive, work, make love. If your thyroid gland is sluggish, so are you. You look and feel old and tired. Even if you do make it as far as the bedroom, you go there only to sleep.

You can complain about your weight, eat a low-fat, low-calorie diet and still gain weight because less of your food is burned for energy and more is stored away as fat.

You don't look or feel sexy!

What does this have to do with the food you eat?

Your thyroid gland needs iodine. Not many land-based foods contain this mineral but seafood and sea vegetables are loaded with the energy-giving nutrient. So, a succulent fish dish seasoned with a sprinkle of kelp powder may be the difference between bed and being "bedded."

From the Sea

Chili Fish Sticks

1 1/2 pounds fish steaks (swordfish, halibut, tuna)
1 tablespoon olive oil
1 onion, sliced
2 green chili peppers, chopped
1 pound can Italian tomatoes (use 1/2 and save the rest)
1/2 tablespoon oregano
Pinch fresh pepper

Coat the bottom of a large casserole with the oil. Put in the onions, garlic, and chilies and cook gently for about five minutes.

Add tomatoes, herbs, and pepper. Season the fish steaks and place them on top of the mixture in the casserole.

Cook over medium heat on top of the stove for about twenty minutes, basting frequently. Turn the steaks once to make sure they are fully cooked.

Serve with fried bananas and broccoli with garlic bread and wine.

How Far Would You Go for Sexual Pleasure? Would You Risk Your Life?

Thankfully, most people find recipes, like those in this book, stimulating enough, but upwards of 100 people a year play the game of sex-or-death... and lose! Not from any recipe we offer but from a seafood that guarantees sexual excitement.

Off the coast of Japan there swims a blowfish called the FUGU. Just behind the head is a delectable, sexually stimulating portion of meat. But the rest of the fish is pure poison and the part that is closest to the edible portion is full of the most potent nerve poison known to man. Cooks are trained for three years in the preparation and serving of FUGU, in how to separate the edible from the poisonous. However, even the best can miss.

Does the excitement of death contribute to the sexual effect? Will the diner walk to the bed of his beloved . . . or be carried to the cemetery? FUGU is not for the fainthearted!

Fish With Fennel

Fennel adds a "licorice" taste which improves the flavor of fish. It also is good for your eyes and ears and was presumed to be an aphrodisiac because of the two ball-like roots.

2 to 3 pounds of fish
(Bass, red snapper, whole or in chunks)
1 1/2 pounds tomatoes
1/2 teaspoon ground ginger
Pinch saffron
1 chopped clove or garlic
1/4 teaspoon dried ground chilies
Freshly ground pepper
Juice of 1 lemon
3 pitted green olives
1 head of fennel, sliced
Fresh coriander as garnish

Marinade

(1 cup fresh coriander leaves, as garnish)
4 cloves of garlic, peeled
2 tablespoons apple cider vinegar
Juice of one lemon
1 tablespoon ground cumin
1/2 teaspoon crushed chilies
2 tablespoons olive oil or canola oil
Cayenne pepper to taste

Combine the ingredients in a blender and blend until well-mixed and smooth.

To make fish with fennel — wash fish, pat dry and marinate for at least one hour.

Peel and seed the tomatoes. Place in saucepan with the ginger, saffron, garlic, chilies, oil and pepper. Simmer gently, stirring frequently until you have a purée.

Add the lemon and olives and set aside.

Arrange the fennel slices across the bottom of a heavy casserole. Place the fish on the fennel and pour on the remaining marinade and the purée. Cook on the top of the stove over medium-low heat for a half-hour, or, if you prefer, bake for 45 minutes at 350°.

Garnish with coriander.

Broiled Oysters

Buy big oysters, fresh and sweet-smelling.

Remove the oysters from their shells and season them with a mixture of minced thyme, grated nutmeg, grated bread and a pinch of salt.

Clean their shells and put them on a plate.

Put the oysters back in their shells with a small piece of sweet butter on top.

Heat them in broiler until their liquor bubbles low.

When crisp, add a drop of wine and cook a minute longer.

Sprinkle them with grated nutmeg and enjoy.

Oyster Cocktail

Season the oysters with a few chopped shallots, one tablespoon of wine vinegar, 1/2 tablespoon of tomato sauce, a few drops of Worcestershire sauce and a little chopped parsley.

Mussels à la Marinière

Take about four dozen fresh mussels, wash them, brush them, scrub them well.

Put them into a saucepan over a good fire with a little butter, some chopped shallots, parsley and chervil.

As soon as the mussels open they are done.

Lower the heat, pour a glass of white wine over them and a sprinkle of pepper.

Serve at once with some freshly chopped parsley sprinkled over them.

Oysters and Bacon

This is delicious!

Shell the oysters, clean them well.

Wrap each oyster in a thin slice of lean bacon and secure the bacon in place with a toothpick.

Put them in a baking tin and into a hot oven until the bacon is cooked.

Serve with a sprinkle of chopped parsley over them and a drop of Worcestershire sauce.

Make a lot because they are good.

Oyster Fricassee

Get a stewing pan and put a little butter, a slice of ham, a sliced onion and minced cloves of garlic in it.

Heat over a low flame till the onion becomes golden.

Add a tablespoon of flour, a glass of broth and a piece of lemon peel.

Then put scalded oysters in the mixture and let them simmer.

When the oysters are ready, thicken the mixture with the yolks of two eggs, a spoonful of cream and a good stir.

Remove what's left of the ham, the lemon peel and the onion and add the juice of a lemon.

Peppery Crabs

1/2 pound fresh crab meat
2 tablespoons canola oil or olive oil
1 onion, chopped
1 clove of garlic, minced
1 green pepper, chopped
1 1/2 hot chilies, finely chopped
3 tomatoes, peeled and chopped
1 1/2 tablespoons tomato purée

1/4 cup dry sherry
Pinch of pepper
1 tablespoon lime juice
1 tablespoon chopped fresh parsley

Into a heavy skillet put the oil, onion, garlic, peppers, and chilies. Cook until tender.

Add the tomatoes, tomato purée, sherry, and pepper and cook, stirring, for about ten minutes. Put in the lime juice and the crab meat.

Cook over a low heat, covered, for about 3 minutes but do not overcook. Sprinkle with parsley and serve over a bed of white or brown rice with a glass of white wine.

Red Mullets in a Special Shrimp Sauce

One fish is good, two are better!

Sauce
Chopped parsley
Teaspoon of capers
Finely chopped onion
Several shrimps pounded to a pulp
Juice of one lemon
Teaspoon of Dijon mustard

Mix thoroughly, heat in olive oil.

Clean the Red Mullets, put them in melted butter, season with a pinch of salt and pepper then grill them over a slow fire until cooked.

Put the fish on a plate and cover with the sauce.

Serve with French bread and wine.

Voila!

Frogs Legs

Get three dozen frogs' legs.

Wash well and put them into a saucepan with a dozen chopped mushrooms, four chopped shallots, and a tablespoon of good olive oil.

Toss them on a fire for about five minutes, then add a tablespoon of flour, a pinch of salt and pepper and a pinch of nutmeg.

Toss a little more, then add a glass of white wine and six ounces of consommé.

Boil for ten minutes.

Meanwhile, mix the yolks of four eggs with two tablespoons of cream.

Remove the frogs' legs and other ingredients from the fire, add the egg and cream mixture, stirring continually until thoroughly mixed, and serve.

This mixture is thought to be highly aphrodisiac in action.

Hot Scallops

1/2 pound sea scallops
Juice of half a lemon
Medium onion, chopped
2 cloves of garlic, minced
1 1/2 tablespoons canola oil or olive oil
1 1/2 cups Italian tomatoes, chopped with juice
Pinch pepper
1/4 teaspoon hot pepper
1/2 teaspoon fresh rosemary leaves or 1/4 teaspoon dried
1 tablespoon butter, melted
1/2 cup fine bread crumbs, toasted
5 ounces linguini

To make hot scallops:

Marinate the scallops in lemon juice for one hour. Meanwhile, soften the onion and the garlic in some of the oil. Add the tomatoes, pepper, hot pepper, and rosemary.

Simmer gently, uncovered, for twenty minutes.

Dry the scallops on a paper towel, dip into the melted butter and the bread crumbs. Broil, turning once until they are lightly browned.

To make the linguini:

Into 3 quarts of boiling water, put the linguini and cook until al dente. Drain and toss with the remaining oil.

Serve the linguini topped with the scallops and the sauce.

Sesame Sea Bass

2 pounds of sea bass
2 tablespoons tahini
1 clove garlic, peeled
1 green chili, seeded
1 tablespoon canola oil
1 tablespoon light soy sauce
1 tablespoon fresh ginger, minced
Juice of half a lemon
Sprinkle of ground pepper
1 tablespoon fresh thyme leaves
2 scallions, diced
1 tablespoon toasted sesame seeds

Preheat oven to 375°.

Wash fish and towel dry. Put the tahini, garlic, chili, oil, soy sauce, ginger, lemon, and pepper in a blender and mix until you get a purée. Mix in the fresh thyme leaves and spread the mixture over the outside and into the inside of the fish.

Sprinkle the scallions over the fish and bake for 45 minutes or until done.

Sprinkle the sesame seeds over the fish and serve with a white wine, unless you have red wine that you like with the sesame tone.

Cacciucco

This dish is similar to French Bouillabaisse but a little sloppier. Great for the cook who likes to throw things together and have it turn out wonderfully . . .

Usually the following fish are used:

A small eel
Small red mullets
Mussels
Mackerel
Pieces of larger fish

Take about two pounds all together with 1/4 pound of fresh tomatoes, one onion, two garlic cloves, two tablespoons of olive oil, two tablespoons of vinegar, a sprig of thyme, half a dry red pepper, some parsley and a pinch of salt and pepper.

Chop fine the onion, parsley, thyme, garlic, pepper and put them into a saucepan with the oil.

Fry until the onion browns, then add the tomatoes which are cut into small pieces.

Season with salt and pepper and let cook well.

Add the vinegar and a little water if necessary.

Boil for five minutes and strain the liquid.

Put it back on the fire and add the fish.

When the fish is done, add 1/2 tablespoon of oil.

Put some toast in the bottom of a soup tureen and pour the fish and liquid over it.

Serve hot.

Shrimp Paprikash

2 tablespoons shallots
2 tablespoons butter
1 pound of peeled shrimp
Pinch of freshly ground pepper

Cayenne pepper to taste
1 tablespoon Hungarian paprika
1/4 cup heavy cream
1/4 cup sour cream
1/2 tablespoon Dijon mustard
Parsley to garnish

Chop the shallots and soften them in the butter.

Add the shrimp and cook just until they turn pink. Add the pepper, cayenne, and paprika and cook another three minutes.

Put in the creams and the mustard and heat thoroughly but without bringing to a boil. Sprinkle with parsley and serve with brown rice and broccoli.

Mussel Muscles

15–20 mussels
1/2 inch cube of fresh ginger, sliced
4 cloves of garlic, minced
3/4 cup water
2 tablespoons canola or olive oil
1 onion, chopped
1 hot, green chili, sliced finely
1/2 teaspoon ground turmeric
1/2 teaspoon ground cumin
Half coconut, grated finely

Wash mussels well, remove beards, discard any with shells open or partly open.

Put garlic and ginger into blender, add 1/4 cup water and blend until smooth.

Heat the oil in a large pot over a medium flame. Sauté onions until translucent. Put in paste from the blender, chilies, turmeric, and cumin. Stir well and fry for one minute. Add the coconut and 1/2 cup of water and bring to a boil.

Add the mussels, mix and bring to boil once again. Lower heat slightly and let mussels steam 5 to 10 minutes or until they open up (discard any that don't open at this point) . . . then serve at once.

Baked Eels

Get 1 1/2 pounds of eels.

Put 2 ounces of a good olive oil in a casserole and heat.

When hot, sprinkle in a teaspoonful of flour, stirring constantly, and add a pinch of grated nutmeg, a handful of parsley and a pinch of salt and pepper, plus some chopped mushrooms.

Add the eels.

Pour in a glass of white wine and a small glass of brandy.

Cover the casserole and transfer it to a moderate oven.

Bake until done.

If you like eels, this is a delicious dish!

Eels From Athens

Start with some good fish stock, a few mushrooms, one tablespoon of vinegar, one tablespoon of French Dijon mustard, one of anchovy sauce and a little chopped parsley.

Mix all of them together in a saucepan and let simmer for about fifteen minutes.

Wash the eels well, dry them with some toweling and cut into small pieces.

Flour them lightly and fry them in olive oil.

When fried and done put them on a plate and cover them with the sauce.

Serve piping hot.

Hot & Dark Shrimp

1 pound shrimp, peeled, deveined, washed and patted dry
1 onion, chopped

2 cloves of garlic
1/2 fresh ginger, chopped
1 cup of water
2 tablespoons canola oil or olive oil
1/2 teaspoon ground cardamom
1/2 teaspoon ground cinnamon
1 bay leaf
1/2 teaspoon ground cumin
1/2 teaspoon ground coriander
1 tomato, peeled and finely chopped
2 tablespoons plain yogurt
1/4 teaspoon ground turmeric
1 teaspoon cayenne pepper
1 tablespoon finely chopped coriander (fresh) (Optional)

Put the onion, garlic, ginger, and 1 1/2 tablespoons of water into a blender and blend into a purée.

Heat the oil over a medium flame and add cinnamon, cardamom, and bay leaf. Stir for 5 seconds. Then add purée and stir and fry for about 5 minutes or until the mixture turns light brown.

Put in the cumin and coriander, stir fry for 30 seconds, then add the tomato and incorporate 1 tablespoon yogurt. Slowly stir in the rest of the yogurt, then put in the turmeric and the cayenne pepper. Add the rest of the water and the shrimp and bring to a boil over a medium-high flame. Stir and cook for about 5 minutes or until the sauce thickens.

Do not overcook — serve at once.

Cuttlefish and Rice

Clean well half a pound of cuttlefish, keeping the little bag with the ink separate.

Cut the cuttlefish into small pieces and let them soak in water for half an hour.

Some Sea-Spawned Aphrodisia

It is said that one of the most powerful of Chinese aphrodisiac recipes is that of *Bird Nest Soup*, prepared from the nests of the sea-swallow (salangane). It is strongly spiced and, so far as taste is concerned, is not dissimilar to the potage à la bisque d'ecrevisses (crayfish soup) of the French. The aphrodisiac effect is difficult to deny although Europeans have often wondered how a bird's nest can be used for the production of a soup.

It is simply explained, although few people live near enough to a colony of sea-swallows to exploit the idea. The nests are made from an edible seaweed, the leaves being stuck together by the spawn of fish. The fish spawn is extremely rich in phosphorus which has a powerful action, increasing both desire and ability. Too much can contribute to overexcitation but not to worry, it's very expensive.

The poor man has a substitute in his *nuoc-man*. Our boys in Vietnam had the opportunity to sample this version of the aphrodisiac soup. It is an extract from rotten fish, and the preparation is similar to that of cod-liver oil. It tastes somewhat like this well-known fish oil, and also contains a high percentage of phosphorus. *Nuoc-man* is heightened in flavor by the use of copious amounts of garlic and pimiento, additional aphrodisiacs.

And then there's caviar. Fish eggs (roe) from any fish is fine, but when we think of caviar we usually mean the roe of the sturgeon. In one hundred grams of caviar there are three hundred and thirty five milligrams of bioactive phosphorus available for sexual metabolic activity.

Chop finely one big onion and two cloves of garlic plus half a red pimiento.

Place three tablespoons of olive oil in a saucepan and brown the vegetables.

When the onion is brown, toss in the fish and let it cook until it is yellow.

Add half a pound of chopped spinach and let the whole thing cook for half an hour.

Add a pound of rice and the little bag from the fish which contains the ink. Stir well with a wooden spoon to make sure the bag breaks and the ink is well distributed.

Add hot water, little by little, with a bit of tomato sauce.

When the rice is cooked and all of the water has been absorbed, serve hot with some Italian wine.

Hot & Spicy Cod Steaks

2 cod steaks, about 1 pound each
1/4 teaspoon cayenne powder
1/4 teaspoon ground turmeric
4 tablespoons canola or olive oil
1/2 teaspoon whole fennel seeds
1/2 teaspoon whole black pepper seeds
1 onion, finely chopped
1 clove of garlic, chopped
1 teaspoon ground cumin seeds
1/2 pound can of tomatoes, chopped
1/2 teaspoon ground cumin seeds

Wash fish steaks and pat dry with paper towels. Rub them on both sides with cayenne and turmeric and set aside for 30 minutes.

Heat 2 tablespoons of oil in a saucepan over medium heat. Add fennel and mustard seeds. When the mustard seeds pop (only a few seconds) add onions and garlic. Stir until the onions turn light brown, then add the cumin and a bit of cayenne. Stir quickly and add the tomatoes and their sauce, then the cumin and bring to a boil.

Cover, turn heat to low and cook gently for 15 minutes. Preheat oven to 350°, put the rest of the oil into a large, non-stick frying pan and heat over a medium-high flame. When hot, put in the fish steaks and brown on both sides. Do not cook the fish through. Put the fish in a baking dish and pour the cooked tomato sauce over them. Bake, uncovered for 15 minutes or until the fish is done.

Non-Quite Sushi

There are times you may want a cool-hot appetizer on a summer afternoon . . .

2 pounds red snapper, extremely fresh and filleted
Juice of 3 lemons
1/2 cup canola oil or olive oil
4 fresh chilies, chopped
2 tablespoons fresh thyme
2 tablespoons fresh parsley, chopped
Freshly ground black pepper
Sprinkle coarse salt
1/2 cup freshly grated coconut

Slice the fillets into 2 by 3 inch pieces. Place the fish in a bowl and cover with the lemon juice. Let stand for about three hours or until the fish turns opaque.

Combine the rest of the ingredients and toss the fish in the mixture. Serve well chilled.

Pescado P.R.

Fish prepared the Island way:

1 to 2 pounds of red snapper
1 onion, sliced
1 green pepper, sliced
1/2 pimiento, sliced

1 clove of garlic, minced
1/4 teaspoon black pepper
1 tablespoon apple cider vinegar
1 tablespoon tomato paste
1 bay leaf
1/2 cup water
4 ounces of canola oil or olive oil

Place everything, except the fish and the oil in a small pot. Heat to a boil then lower flame and simmer, covered, for ten minutes.

In a skillet, sauté fish until almost done. Drain off the oil. Cover fish with the vegetable mixture and cook an additional 5 to 7 minutes, or until done.

Serve with some wine or a glass of ice-cold beer to balance the flavors.

Coriander Mackerel

Mackerel is one of the fishes which contain oils helpful to circulation, but it's hard to prepare mackerel so it doesn't have a "fishy" taste. This dish makes mackerel a delight and provides energy for after-meal sport.

1 pound mackerel fillet
3 tablespoons fresh, green coriander, finely chopped
1 hot green chili, finely chopped
1 tablespoon lemon juice
Freshly ground black pepper
2 tablespoons butter

Combine the coriander, chili, lemon juice and pepper in a bowl. Mix well. Rub the mixture all over the fillet. Let stand for 45 minutes.

Heat the broiler. Put the fillet in the broiling tray and dot with half the butter. Broil 4 inches from the flame for 5 minutes. Turn the fish over, dot with the remaining butter and broil for 4 minutes or until golden brown.

This fish dish will make any guest sit up and take notice. Invite your guest into the kitchen as a participant. It's a nice prelude for things to come.

Fish Fillets in Paper

1 1/2 pounds fish fillets (striped bass, weakfish, flounder, bluefish, fluke)
2 tablespoons and a bit of canola oil or olive oil
1 cup onions, sliced
1 cup mushrooms, sliced
1 cup canned, drained tomatoes
1 bay leaf
1/2 teaspoon dried thyme
1/4 teaspoon hot red pepper flakes
Freshly ground pepper and a pinch of coarse salt

Preheat oven to 350°.

Cut fillets into four pieces of equal size and length.

Cut four pieces of parchment or foil about 24 inches long and 12 inches wide.

Heat 2 tablespoons of oil in a skillet and add the onion, garlic, green pepper and mushrooms. Cook, stirring, until the onions and the peppers are wilted. Add the tomatoes, bay leaf and thyme, plus pepper, salt and pepper flakes to taste.

Brush the paper lightly with oil. Place one fillet in the center of the paper and spoon one quarter of the tomato mixture over it. Fold and seal the edges of the paper as airtight as possible. Do the rest of the fillets the same way.

Arrange the fillets on a baking sheet and bake in the oven for ten minutes.

Remove from oven and transfer to dinner plates. Enjoy along with a chilled white wine and crusty French bread.

From the Pasture and the Chicken Coop

Chinese-Style Stir-Fried Spicy Beef

1 pound butt steak
3 tablespoons dry sherry
2 tablespoons lite soy sauce
3 tablespoons sesame oil
2 cloves of garlic, minced
2 tablespoons fresh ginger, minced
3 scallions, chopped
1/2 teaspoon fresh pepper
Pinch coarse salt

Slice the butt steak against the grain into thin strips.

Combine the sherry, soy sauce, 2 tablespoons of sesame oil, garlic and ginger and marinate the meat in the mixture for one hour.

Heat the remaining oil in a skillet. Stir-fry the beef, including the marinade, for 2 to 3 minutes with the scallions. Do not overcook or the meat will be tough. Serve with brown rice and a cup of Saki warmed to body temperature.

Indoor Bar-B-Q with Spicy Moroccan Meatballs

1 pound ground beef or lamb or a mix of the two
1 onion, grated
1/2 teaspoon ground cumin seeds
1 teaspoon paprika
1/4 cup chopped parsley, fresh
1 sprig fresh mint, chopped
1/4 teaspoon ground cinnamon

Pinch coarse salt
Pinch fresh pepper

Mix the meat and the rest of the ingredients in a bowl and let stand to develop flavor. After one hour, wet your hands and form the mixture into oblong patties. Wrap the patties around long skewers and grill them over high heat.

Spiced Beef

1 pound of beef steak
1/2 tablespoon coriander seeds
1 fresh chili, chopped
1/2 teaspoon turmeric
1/3 tablespoon fresh ginger, chopped
1 clove of garlic
1 onion, chopped
2 macadamia nuts
2 tablespoons canola oil or olive oil
1/2 cup coconut milk
1/2 tablespoon brown sugar
1 tablespoon grated lemon peel
Pinch of coarse salt
Pinch of fresh pepper

In a blender, place the coriander, chili, turmeric, ginger, garlic, onion, and macadamia nuts. Add a bit of oil to ease the blending and combine until smooth.

In a heavy skillet, place a tablespoon of oil and the spice mixture and heat until thickened. Then add the coconut milk, sugar, lemon peel, salt and pepper and bring to a boil. Remove from heat.

Cut the beef into 1-inch cubes and thread onto small skewers. Grill under broiler brushing generously with the sauce. Cook for two to three minutes then turn. Serve over brown rice with the rest of the sauce.

Peppercorn Steak

This steak bites back. Very stimulating!

Use a mortar and pestle to crush the peppercorns. A mill will grind them too finely for this recipe. If you don't have a mortar and pestle, put the peppercorns in a cloth and bang them with a hammer. If you don't have a hammer, borrow one from the neighbor.

1 to 2 pounds boneless steak (fillet mignon or sirloin)
1/2 cup black peppercorns
1 tablespoon butter
1 tablespoon canola oil
1/4 cup brandy
1/2 cup heavy cream
Coarse salt to taste

(This is not a dish for the cholesterol-watcher.)

Trim the fat from the steaks and crush the peppercorns. With the heel of your hand press the peppercorns firmly into both sides of the meat.

Heat the butter and oil in a heavy frying pan and cook the steaks over high heat. Remove to a warm plate.

Remove the frying pan from the heat and add the brandy. Put the pan back on the heat and bring the brandy to a boil, taking care that it does not flare up. Cook for 2 minutes which is enough to boil off the alcohol, scraping up the cooking juices. Add the cream, heat through, season with a pinch of salt, then pour the mixture over the steaks and serve at once.

Who could resist this dish?

Baked Pork Roast

2 1/2 pound pork roast
1/4 cup canola oil or olive oil
2 medium onions, chopped
2 cloves of garlic, minced

1/2 teaspoon coriander seeds, crushed
1 bay leaf
1 pound tomatoes, peeled
1/2 cup tarragon vinegar
1/2 teaspoon crushed red chili pepper
1/2 tablespoon chili powder
Pinch coarse salt
Pinch pepper

Heat the oil in a saucepan and sauté the onions and garlic until soft.

Add all the remaining ingredients except the pork and simmer gently for about 45 minutes, covered.

Trim the roast pork in a roasting pan and bake in a preheated oven at 350° for about two hours, basting with the sauce.

The sauce will be dark and delicious. Dark red wine is delicious with this dish although ice-cold beer goes equally well.

A Mint of Chopped Lamb

Enough for 3, if that's your pleasure:

1 medium onion, chopped
4 garlic cloves, peeled and chopped
Small piece of ginger, peeled and chopped
2 tablespoons of water
1 tablespoon ground cumin
2 teaspoons ground coriander
1/2 teaspoon turmeric
1/2 teaspoon cayenne pepper
2 tablespoons olive oil
2 cardamom pods
1 pound ground lamb
Sprinkle of salt
1/2 cup chopped mint leaves, fresh
1 tablespoon lemon juice

Mix the onion, garlic, ginger and water in a blender and blend until you get a smooth paste. Add the cumin, coriander, turmeric and cayenne and blend for 10 seconds.

Heat the oil in a 10 inch frying pan over high heat. When hot, add the cardamom. Turn heat to medium and put in the spice mixture. Stir and heat for 3 minutes. Add a bit of water if the mixture sticks.

Put in the ground meat and stir until all of the pink is gone. Add the salt and mix. Cover and let cook for 1/2 hour. Add the mint leaves, lemon juice and bring to simmer. Remove cardamom pods before serving.

Lamb Sticks

Like long, spicy meatballs, guaranteed stimulating!

1 pound ground lamb
1 inch ginger, peeled and ground
1 teaspoon ground cumin
1 teaspoon ground coriander
1 teaspoon ground cloves
1/4 teaspoon ground cinnamon
1/8 teaspoon grated nutmeg
1/8 teaspoon ground black pepper
1/4 teaspoon cayenne pepper
Sprinkle salt
3 tablespoons plain yogurt
4 tablespoons canola oil
1 bay leaf
4 ounces of water

Combine the lamb, ginger, coriander, cumin, cloves, cinnamon, nutmeg, peppers, salt and yogurt in a bowl and mix well. Wet your hands with cold water and make sausages from the mixture. Heat the oil in a non-stick fry pan. Throw in the bay leaf and place the sausages in the oil, single layer. Fry until lightly brown on all sides. Add water and let simmer for a half-hour, turning the sausages every so often. It's done when all of the water has left the fry pan. Lift the sausages out of the pan with a slotted spoon, leaving the fat behind.

Spicy-Hot Baked Chicken

1 teaspoon ground cumin
2 teaspoons paprika
1 teaspoon cayenne pepper
1 teaspoon ground turmeric
1 teaspoon black pepper
Sprinkle salt
2 cloves of garlic, mashed
2 pounds of chicken pieces, no skin
1 1/2 tablespoons canola oil

Mix the cumin, paprika, cayenne, turmeric, pepper, salt, garlic with three tablespoons of lemon juice. Rub the mixture over the chicken parts, covering everything. Put the chicken pieces in a shallow baking tray and let stand in a cool place for 3 hours. Cover with plastic wrap to prevent drying.

Preheat oven to 400 degrees. Brush the chicken tops with oil. Bake for 20 minutes. Turn over and bake for another 20 to 25 minutes or until tender. Baste with the drippings every 5 minutes.

Get some white wine and some tasty bread and eat this spicy chicken with your fingers. If you don't like it too spicy, cut down on the amount of cayenne pepper, but don't leave it out altogether.

Meatballs with Eggplant Sauce

2 pounds ground chuck or lean lamb
1/4 cup pine nuts
1/4 cup white raisins
Sprinkle of sea salt
1 tablespoon paprika
1 teaspoon oregano

2 eggs
1/4 cup flour
1/4 cup olive oil

In a bowl, combine meat, nuts, raisins, salt, paprika, oregano, and eggs. Mix lightly with a fork.

Wet your hands and shape into about 24 meatballs. Roll lightly in the flour. Lightly brown them all over in 1/4 cup oil, then turn up heat until all browned, then lower heat and cook covered for fifteen minutes more.

To make the sauce:

1/4 cup canola oil or olive oil
1 cup chopped onion
1 eggplant, pared and cut into 1/2 inch cubes
1 can Italian plum tomatoes, undrained
Sprinkle of salt
1/2 teaspoon ground cumin
1/2 teaspoon ground coriander

In a 5 quart Dutch oven, sauté onions until tender in 1/4 cup oil. Add eggplant and cook over medium heat, stirring frequently. After five minutes stir in remaining ingredients. Bring to boil, simmer covered about half an hour.

Arrange meatballs on a heated dish, spoon sauce over them and serve with wine and garlic bread.

Liver Loaf

1 1/2 slices of bread, in pieces
1 onion, minced
2 large garlic cloves, minced
1/2 cup parsley
2 tablespoons canola oil
1 1/4 pounds liver, remove skin and veins and cut coarsely
3 tablespoons flour
Sprinkle of sea salt

1/2 teaspoon black pepper
1 teaspoon oregano
1 teaspoon basil
1 cup water

Crumble bread into a blender and add the onion, garlic and parsley with enough water to cover. Blend until you have a fine mixture. Strain and sauté until soft.

Put all ingredients into the blender and blend at high speed. Pack into a baking pan. Put a strip of bacon on top and bake at 325 degrees for 1 1/2 hours.

Sour Grapes

"....if she be not for me then what care I for whom she be."

Elias Ashmole, a seventeenth century English alchemist wrote the following verse upon being turned down by a lady of his choice because he was unable to repeat the act of love as often as the lady would have him do. The impossibility led him to wonder about other things he couldn't do:

I asked philosophy how I should
Have of her the thing I would;
She answered me when I was able
To make the water malleable;
Or else the way if I could find
To measure out a yard of wind,
Then shalt thou have thine own desire,
When thou can'st weigh an ounce of fire,
Unless that thou can'st do these three,
Content thyself, thou gets not me.

Perfumes of Love — Aromatherapy

Plants and flowers can add to a seductive mood with color and sheer beauty, but there is another plant gift that can create an actual sexual longing. That gift is the oil the plant uses to make its individual scent.

Aromatherapy is the use of essential oils from plants to revitalize and enhance health and beauty as well as the desire to make love.

We have experienced aromatherapy all of our lives, but never called it by its name. Every time we peeled an orange, put a carnation in our lapel or hair, or washed our face with a mint-scented soap we have utilized this new-old science.

Essential oils are not greasy and are prepared from plants by steam distillation for the most part. This technique involves placing the fresh plant in some kind of a vessel and introducing steam. The steam and the scent-producing parts of the plant rise from the vessel and are then cooled. The insoluble oil is taken off the top of the mixture, leaving a water-soluble extract called a hydrosol.

Oil from citrus fruits can be cold-pressed from the peel but most oils from flowers are extracted with a solvent which is then driven off to leave the absolute oil behind. Aromatherapy oils differ from most scents available by being completely natural. Synthetic oils may appear to smell the same, but they don't have the same therapeutic effect. This sounds strange but it has been proven during experiments with the E.E.G. machine which measures brain waves. The people involved in the experiment inhaled apple blossom scent from nature and a man-made apple blossom perfume. The volunteers could not tell the difference, but their brain waves showed different reactions when one or the other was smelled.

Essential oils can be applied to the body, used to scent a room, placed in the bath or applied to a pillow. The use of these scents are included because lovemaking is stimulated by the release of certain neurochemicals in the brain. These neurochemicals or neurotransmitters are the result of the food you eat and when you eat it. The same neurochemicals can be stimulated by certain scents.

Why Is This So?

The smell area of the brain (the olfactory area) neighbors the sex area and is tied to the more "primitive" area of self-preservation and tribe preservation. Smell plays an enormous part in the sexual behavior of animals and, although we do not think of ourselves as animals, we share many traits since we are inhabitants of the same planet.

Neurochemicals such as *noradrenaline,* the aggressive and sexual chemical, can be triggered by stimulating oils. Others like *endorphins* and *enkephalins,* are partly what make us feel quietly euphoric.

So, after the tastes and smells of your carefully formulated meal have begun the neurochemical process of sexual stimulation, the application or use of aromatherapy is a double-barrelled shot to the same area. And not only to him. The neurochemicals also influence her.

Smelling a flower makes you feel good inside and aromatherapy has the same effect. Then, from the initial like/dislike response to the odor, an emotional response will be invoked in both individuals. The stimulating oils relieve depression and lead into aggressive activity. The evocative power of odors have been known since primitive times and aromatics have been widely used in love potions and aphrodisiacs for centuries.

Feeling good and feeling sexually aroused are linked, although different. Euphoric essential oils such as clary sage and ylang-ylang gain a deep access to our nervous systems because we do not block them.

Essential oils can be purchased in health food stores and are well worth the price. This is not to say that perfumes are not pleasant, but for a sexual campaign we prefer the real thing.

Consider the use of any of the following for romantic purposes:

Clary sage, ylang-ylang, rose, jasmine, patchouli, sandalwood, and linden blossom.

To make an aphrodisiac massage oil,

Mix:

5 drops of jasmine
4 drops of rose
10 drops of sandalwood
2 drops of bergamot
in 2 ounces of a fresh vegetable oil

Rose Perfume

4 drops rose
10 drops sandalwood
2 drops germanium
2 drops rosewood
in 10 ml of jojoba

Jasmine Perfume

2 drops jasmine
10 drops rosewood
5 drops ylang-ylang
in 10 ml jojoba

Whale Wax and Potency

Cardinal Richelieu fathered a child when he was 85. He thought his reheightened ability was the result of fish stew and chocolate bonbons laced with whale wax.

Whale wax (*ambre gris*) is 80% cholesterol, which is one reason to avoid it. The other reason is that we know it in modern terms as ambergris and it originates in the intestines of the sperm whale.

Either apply to strategic points on your body or put a few drops in a tepid bath, swish the water around and relax in the tub for ten minutes. Pat dry, then let the heat of the kitchen release the subtle aromas.

You may not have time to eat!

Making erotic perfumes is a lot like cooking. You read the recipe, get the ingredients and mix. Some perfumes are to be mixed with bath water, some are burned, and others are to be mixed in food. Here are some examples taken from ancient books:

In the Bath Water

Use one teaspoon of the final mixture:

40 grains of powdered incense
8 grains powdered musk
44 grains of myrtle
7 grains of powdered camphor
40 grains of powdered savory flowers

Mix all of the ingredients and place in a bottle containing one pint of rosewater.

Let stand for 48 hours, then filter and add three ounces of rectified alcohol (a good vodka will do) as a preservative.

This concoction acts powerfully on the brain and the sexual parts.

For Burning in an Ashtray

Use the same ingredients, minus the alcohol and the rosewater. Add 20 grains of gum arabic and mix well in a mortar. A tiny amount about the size of a pea can be burned in an incense burner.

Perfume for Food

The following is intended to be used with ten ounces of meat or fish:

45 grains of curcuma
75 grains of pimento (allspice)
45 grains of fenugreek
30 grains of cumin
30 grains of pepper
30 grains of mustard
2/3 ounce of coriander
1 1/2 ounces of onion
1 ounce of tamarind pulp

This is an authentic Indian dish designed to strengthen the genetic senses and the memory.

But only the authenticity is guaranteed!

Which Fragrance Is You?

- Glamorous
- Mysterious
- Exciting
- Sensuous
- Exotic

Words with the power to evoke images. Words that have become almost synonymous with beauty. Small wonder these words are used to describe the effect of scent on the senses.

The power of words and the human sense of smell is such that it almost becomes a puzzle: did the word evoke the scent or the scent evoke the word?

Mysterious . . . the Far East and the odor of sandalwood.

Exotic . . . South Seas Islands and a beautiful wahine with flowers in her hair.

Sensuous . . . Satin sheets and a whiff of a warm, heady aroma.

And it works both ways.

A hint of a certain scent will often remind us of another time, another place, an exciting, romantic situation, a never-to-be-forgotten summer evening, or that very special person.

Most fragrances fall into one of the special basic types, according to their chemical compositions:

- **Oriental** fragrances use musk, civet, and ambergris as fixatives to produce a sultry, exotic, often heady aroma.
- **Spicy** fragrances combine pungent ingredients like cinnamon, clove ginger, vanilla, and spicy flowers such as carnation.
- **Fruity** blends usually have a citrus base and a hint of the refreshing scent of orange, lemon, apricot, peach, tangerine, with a touch of grapefruit.
- **Floral Bouquets** are a blend of a variety of flowers, with no one scent predominating.
- **Single Florals** have the dominant note of one flower, such as rose, gardenia, jasmine, or lily of the valley.
- **Woodsy-mossy** fragrances are a mixture of rosewood, sandalwood, cedarwood and balsam, combined with ferns and herbs. The result can be reminiscent of the fresh, outdoorsy aroma of a forest.

Many people are individuals and reject the idea that commercially prepared perfumes and colognes suit their personality. They prefer to seek out their own aroma. If you are one of those individuals, AROMATHERAPY is designed for you. You can make your own scent by choosing an essential oil or two and mixing them with vodka.

A fragrant cologne can be made by adding 4 drops oil of lavender, 4 drops oil of rosemary, and 1 drop tincture of ambergris to one-half pint of vodka. Shake well, then let it age in a dark place for two weeks.

Sexual Regeneration and Advice to the Aging

Through the ages, men have sought for sexual stimulants in the vegetable kingdom, the animal kingdom, and the wildest combinations of insects and animal organs thinkable. When a particular item performed as desired, it was remembered and passed on from generation to generation. If it didn't work it was forgotten.

The best known stimulants in the vegetable kingdom are: spices of all kinds, mints, cresses, celery, artichoke, asparagus, nutmeg, pimento (allspice), thyme, clove, vanilla beans, saffron, ginseng, salep (dried orchid tuber), truffles, agaric (a mushroom, poisonous in large quantities), morels and several other types of mushroom.

In the animal kingdom (fish and shellfish): lobster, crawfish, shrimp, mollusks, oysters, clams and other bivalves, caviar and roe.

When feeling deficient in the sex department, make sure that your nutrition is at its highest level. Eat seafood, eggs, truffles, lentils, meats — trimmed of fat but strengthened with spices.

Pine nuts, hazel nuts, pistachio nuts, warmed in the oven can be invigorating.

In 1926 the eminent Dutch gynecologist, Th. Van de Velde, published a classic on sexual technique which included a section on erotic cookery. He states that a plentiful diet assists sexual activity while a frugal diet — particularly what is known as underfeeding — leads to a diminution and inhibition of this function. He stresses the value of meat and lists eggs as stimulants and restoratives. He recommends milk-rice dishes, beetroots, carrots, turnips, crayfish soup (which he compares to Chinese bird's nest soup for its aphrodisiac ability), celery, cinnamon, pepper and ginger. And, he says calf's brains tastefully cooked may be of value because of the lecithin content.

Another medical authority, Dr. William J. Robinson, in an exhaustive volume dealing with impotence and frigidity, devotes space to diet. The patient should eat eggs, oysters, raw and cooked meat and fish. He considers saffron, pepper, mustard, cardamom, cinnamon, nutmeg and ginger as having an undoubted effect on stimulating the libido.

From the Vatsyayana on, many voices have been raised in favor of the erotic virtues of garlic. Food heavily flavored with this herb has been a favorite aphrodisiac over the centuries . . . but both people must partake at the same time.

Brillat-Savarin pointed out that a sauté of truffles excites a power, and is a positive aphrodisiac.

Aphrodisiacs are often written about, but can they really jumpstart your sexual inclinations? Volumes of information have been written about alcohol, oysters, ginseng, coffee, powdered rhinoceros horn, ground up beetles and the bark of an African tree. Some sexual stimulants have been proven worthy of their salt, although not rhinoceros horn — the poor beasts have been hunted almost to extinction in the search for instant lust. However, the proper choice of menu *will* add extra passion and luster to otherwise routine lovemaking. In addition, some age-old ideas actually promise to reexcite lost libido!

Oysters Excite More Than the Taste Buds

Scientists scoffed at the idea that they were a virility food until nutritionists showed they contain large mounts of the trace mineral zinc. Zinc is essential for male sexual functioning, and diets deficient in the mineral result in low sperm count and low contact with females. A meal of oysters is no guarantee of great sex, but they will enhance a sexual mood.

Ginseng

Ginseng is an herb that has been venerated in the Orient for centuries. Chinese and Koreans, in particular, believe that it stimulates the ability for intimate congress.

American scientists were skeptical so they tested ginseng on mice. They found that it does excite sexual activity. Did they try it on themselves? If they did, they didn't release a report.

Ginseng is available in many health food stores in tablet or liquid form.

Caffeine in Your Coffee?

If your Don Juan gets sleepy after dinner and heads for the sofa, change your menu and finish the meal with a strong cup of coffee. Caffeine does more than keep your lover awake. University of Michigan urologist Ananias Diokno, M.D. found that coffee drinkers were considerably more sexually active than non-coffee drinkers.

Alcohol

William Shakespeare wrote in Macbeth that "alcohol provokes the desire, but takes away the performance." So, one or two drinks with dinner will ignite the spark, but any more inhibits erections in men and impairs the sexual response in women.

Wellbutrin

In my opinion, aphrodisiacs exist in food and in many plants (see Part One of this book). However, your doctor may choose to prescribe a prescription drug made by Burroughs Welcome. It didn't begin as a sexual stimulant. It began as an antidepressant, but unlike most antidepressants, it didn't dampen the libido. To the contrary, according to T.L. Crenshaw, M.D., of San Diego, it returns dysfunctional men and women to levels of sexual interest that we'd call normal or better.

Ask your M.D. for Wellbutrin. It doesn't work immediately, taking several weeks for improvement, but it truly is a sexual stimulant along with diet, exercise and medical supervision.

Yohimbine

(See also "Yohimbine", page 42)

Yohimbine, from the bark of an African tree, has been reputed to be an aphrodisiac. Scoff no more about folklore! Three studies by Alvero Morales, M.D. of Queen's University in Ontario, Canada, have shown that yohimbine does, indeed, raise erections in some impotent men.

Two prescription drugs containing yohimbine are on the market. One is called Yocon (Palisades Pharmaceuticals) and the other Yohimex (Kramer Laboratories).

A Fourteenth Century Remedy For Impotence

Pound some burdock seeds in a mortar.

Add the left testicle of a three-year old goat, a pinch of hair from the back of a white dog which has been cut on the first day of the new moon.

Place the items in a bottle half-filled with brandy and leave uncorked for exactly 21 days. On the 21st day cook the mixture until it is thickened and add 4 drops of crocodile semen.

Filter and apply to the genitals.

(Since crocodiles were rare in Europe, dog semen was frequently substituted. Even if crocodiles were available, it was a lot easier to obtain the semen from a dog. Crocodiles are not partial to having their genitals handled.)

In any case, this experiment, says the tradition, has always been successful whether dogs or crocodiles are used.

Seduction à la Carte

The *Not For Everyone* Menu Selections!

Shark Fin soup and Bird's Nest soup work for the wistful Chinese, so who are we to exclude receipes which have tantalized Kings and commoners alike.

Fried Brains of Beef

Get some brains
Scald in hot water and clean well
Cut into eight pieces.

Mix together:

Flour
Chopped parsley
Chopped chives
Pinch of allspice

Roll the brains in the mixture until all the pieces are well coated. Heat some olive oil or canola oil in a frying pan and fry the brains until done.

Brains of Veal

Scald two brains of veal in hot water and clean well
Boil some white onions
Make a bouquet garni of:
Half clove of garlic
Sprig of rosemary
Piece of celery
Leaves of parsley

Place the brains in a pan with white wine to cover. Add onions and the bouquet garni and cook until done. When done, remove the brains to a plate and cover with black truffles. Remove the garni, but serve the cooking water and onions over the brains.

Turtle Soup

Take three pounds of turtle
12 cloves
1 onion, diced
1 tablespoon flour
1/2 glass of a good sherry
4 hardboiled eggs
1/2 gallon of water
1/2 teaspoon minced parsley
1/2 teaspoon cayenne pepper
3 tablespoons canola oil
1/2 lemon, sliced

Put the turtle meat up to boil. Add seasoning and cook till tender. Mix flour with canola oil, add lemon and wine. Arrange the sliced hard-boiled eggs around drained turtle meat. Place in serving bowls with strained liquid.

Snakes Madeira

Plunge three large, live diamondbacks into boiling water to remove skins.

Cook in slightly salted water, drain and remove whatever is inside. Cut into bite-sized pieces and place them in a saucepan with some olive oil.

Sauté, then add half pint of Madeira wine.

Boil down until nearly evaporated, then add six egg yolks with a little salt and red pepper.

Stew on a hot flame until tender.

Serve with lemon juice.

(Needless to say, this is a recipe to be handled with care and is not for the average chef.)

Truffled Brains

Get either one calf's brain or two sheep brains.

Clean them well of any red veins.

Put them in a deep pan with some canola or olive oil and brown them on all sides.

When tender and cooked to a turn, place them over a layer of finely sliced truffles.

Before serving, sprinkle them with grated Parmesan cheese.

Curried Kidneys

Fry a minced shallot in a pan with some canola oil until the shallot is nicely browned.

Add a teaspoon of chopped chutney, reduce a bit and strain.

Skin six kidneys, cut in half, remove the cores and dip them in oil. Then roll them in flour seasoned with a little curry powder. Place in a pan and fry until done.

Drain when cooked and serve with some of the chutney mixture.

This dish goes very well with brown rice.

Champagne Kidneys

Cut some kidneys into very thin slices.

Put them into a saucepan over a gentle flame with olive oil, salt, pepper, nutmeg, and sliced mushrooms.

When nearly cooked, add a pinch of flour and a glass of champagne.

Serve with lemon wedges.

Lambs' Ears

About one dozen lambs' ears will be enough for two people.

Take a large handful of sorrel and stew in a chicken broth.

Add some pepper and salt and a pinch of nutmeg.

Add the ears and stew until soft.

Twist the ears and serve on a warmed dish.

Pie of Bull's Testicles

Get four bull's testicles from your local testicle market.

Boil them in salted water.

Strip the membranes that cover them.

Cut them in slices and sprinkle with pepper, salt, cinnamon, and nutmeg.

> *Prepare a mince of lamb's kidney, beef gravy, three slices of lean ham, pinch of chopped marjoram, pinch of thyme, and three chopped cloves.*

Make a regular pie pastry and place it in a pie plate.

Layer as follows:

> *Ham first, then sliced testicles, then sprinkle with the mince.*

Continue making layers until all of the ingredients have been used.

Just before closing the pie add a glass of red wine.

Bake until done and serve.

Sparrows' Brains

Sparrows have always been praised as stimulants for waning sexual prowess.

Aristotle has written: *Propter nimium coitum, vix tertium annum elabuntur.*

Whoever wants to test this should take several brains of male sparrows and half the amount of the brains of pigeons which have not yet begun to fly.

Cut some turnip and a lean carrot in little slices and place the vegetables in a deep pan with half a glass of goat's milk.

Boil till the milk is almost absorbed. Then put in the brains and sprinkle them with powdered clover seeds.

Remove from the flame as soon as dish comes to a boil and serve.

For Sexual Continuity

Organ meats make for better lovers than muscle meats.

Liver is as high in phosphorus as any fish and is a wonderful source of energy-giving B vitamins.

Brains and Sweetbreads (thymus gland) are highly praised. Not only for their protein, vitamins and minerals, but for their high lecithin content. Lecithin is a rich source of phosphorus and the raw material for the manufacture of steroids and sterones, including the male and female hormones.

Snails served Petronius well when the *Satyricon's* hero needed a restorative.

The genitals of many animals have served to boost the potency of many men throughout the ages. Bulls, rams and goats have given their all and were highly recommended by Alexandre Dumas (père) in *Le Grand Dictionnaire de Cuisine.* Calf's testicles were favored in Omero Rompini's *La Cucina dell'Amore.*

In the Far East, tiger's testicles were the choice of kings . . . which accounts for the shortage of tigers today.

Skink (A Reptile Aphrodisiac)

The skink is lauded as a sexual stimulant in many ancient books. Mesue preferred the tails of skink. Tristram speaks of roasted skink.

The problem is not if this recipe works but how to find a fresh skink. However, if you chance to be strolling in Africa or Arabia and come across a skink that is large enough for cooking, this is the way to prepare it.

Fillet the skink along the backbone, soak in beaten eggs, season with a sprinkle of salt, a pinch of cayenne pepper and fry until soft and delicious, using either olive oil or canola oil.

The ancient books do not specify male or female skink and I'm not sure if the average person can tell the difference, so, whatever skink you find is probably as good as the next one.

Vulvae Steriles

Apicius wrote of this dish in the book "Polyteles".

The Ancient Romans praised it to the ceiling for its amatory restimulation.

Horace, Pliny, and Martial were partial to its power.

If you would care to partake of this unusual dish . . .

> *Take that part of a sow, clean it well and marinate in white wine to which is added a chopped onion, a branch of celery, a pinch of fennel, some ground peppercorns, some minced ginger, a pinch of saffron and a sprinkle of salt.*
>
> *Let marinate for three hours.*
>
> *Sprinkle with flour and place in a casserole dish with a tablespoon of olive oil.*
>
> *Let brown on all sides.*
>
> *Use the marinade to moisten it from time to time.*
>
> *When nearly cooked, add the juice of a lemon and an orange and serve hot.*

Garlic Needs a Special Section of its Own

Many people turn up their noses at even the thought of this splendid herb. However, from the *Vatsyayana* to *The Perfumed Garden,* there is considerable faith in the erotic virtues of garlic.

This is what the wily sheik has written:

"There is one spice or condiment of which I hesitate to speak, because it is held in such contempt and disdain in this country. I refer to garlic. There can, however, be no question as to its *pronounced aphrodisiac effect.* In fact it stands at the head of the list. But many of our Anglo-Saxons would prefer their impotence to the alternative of having to eat garlic. The nations, however, who have no such loathing of the bulb of *allium sativum,* the Italians and the Jews, for instance, often make use of garlic as an aphrodisiac; some do it with deliberation, instinctively so to say."

What Is the Mystery Of Garlic?

In the early 1920's, a Russian biologist made a startling study. His name was Alexander Gurvich and he found that if an onion plant's growing tip was pointed at the growing tissue of another onion, the other onion grew twice as fast and twice as large.

He called the energy released by the growing tip *mitogenetic* radiation.

Onions, garlic and all cousins of the lily have been considered to be panaceas since the earliest of times.

Onions and garlic confer vigor upon the eater.

Among the Ancient Greeks, garlic, leeks, and onions were considered to be aphrodisiacs.

Among the Romans, Martial advised, "If your wife is old and your member exhausted, eat onions in plenty."

Sexologist William J. Robinson, after extensive medical tests, was convinced of garlic's pronounced aphrodisiac effect.

And it adds such a good taste to all foods!

The sheik wrote a long time ago but modern studies, although not conceding the aphrodisiac ability, do credit garlic with myriad benefits. Among them: lowering blood cholesterol, killing the virus that causes cold sores, breaking down blood clots that can cause problems in the circulatory system, and helping to neutralize agents that can cause stomach cancer.

Garlic is a leader in the field of medicine but its true kingdom remains in the kitchen.

Here are a few garlic recipes to whet your appetite.

Garlic Chicken

Take 2 pounds boned chicken breasts cut into 1 inch cubes
2 tablespoons olive oil
1 garlic bulb, peeled and crushed
1 teaspoon tarragon
Pinch salt
1/2 teaspoon black pepper
1/2 teaspoon cayenne pepper
1 cup water

Preheat oven to 350°.

Sauté chicken cubes in oil over medium heat for 10 minutes.

Add garlic and stir fry for 4 minutes.

Transfer to a casserole dish.

In a separate dish, mix remaining ingredients and then add to the casserole.

Stir, cover and bake for 30 minutes.

Uncover and bake another 30 minutes or until chicken is tender.

Serve on brown rice.

Garlic and Zucchini

1 garlic bulb, peeled and sliced
2 tablespoons olive oil
1 1/2 pounds zucchini cut into 1/4 inch slices
4 tablespoons vinegar
2 tablespoons cilantro, chopped finely
Pinch salt
1/2 teaspoon black pepper
1/8 teaspoon cayenne pepper

Sauté the garlic in olive oil over medium heat until the garlic slices turn golden brown. Remove garlic with a slotted spoon and set aside.

In the same oil, sauté the zucchini until golden brown, turning once.

Remove and drain on paper towels.

Combine the other ingredients in a bowl and set aside.

Place zucchini on a serving platter and sprinkle the vinegar mixture over the slices.

Top evenly with the garlic and allow to stand for 3 to 4 hours before serving.

Smells delicious and tastes as good as it smells!

Garlic Barbecue Sauce

1 garlic bulb, peeled and crushed
4 tablespoons olive oil
4 tablespoons lemon juice
1/8 teaspoon cayenne pepper

Just put all of the ingredients into a blender and mix thoroughly for one minute.

Mashed Potatoes with Garlic and Pistachios

3 cups mashed potatoes
1/2 garlic bulb, peeled and crushed
1/2 cup shelled pistachios
1 tablespoon olive oil
Pinch salt
1/2 teaspoon black pepper
1/2 teaspoon nutmeg
6 tablespoons water

Place the mashed potatoes in a bowl.

Blend the rest of the ingredients in a blender for one minute.

Thoroughly combine the blended ingredients with the mashed potatoes.

Serve hot.

Roast Garlic for Two

Place twenty large garlic cloves, peeled but otherwise whole, in a small casserole with 3 tablespoons of sweet butter and a tablespoon of canola oil, and a pinch of salt and pepper.

Bake at 350° for at least 20 minutes.

Stir and baste often.

Both of you sit down on the sofa with this dish, one glass each of red wine.

Oh my!

Chicken Garlic Noodle Soup

2 pounds of chicken bones with a little meat
1 cup fine noodles
3 cloves of garlic, peeled and mashed
1 tablespoon chopped fresh cilantro
Sprinkle salt
1/4 teaspoon black pepper

1/4 teaspoon thyme
1/4 teaspoon nutmeg
1/8 teaspoon cayenne pepper
1 tablespoons chopped green onion
1 tablespoon finely chopped mint

Put the bones in a pot and cover with 3 inches of water. Bring to boil and cover. Cook over medium heat for 2 hours. Strain to remove bones. Add water to make 4 cups of liquid. Add remaining ingredients except onion and mint.

Bring to boil and cover. Cook 25 minutes over medium heat. Remove from heat, add onions and mint and serve with crusty Italian bread.

Garlic Potatoes

2 pounds potatoes
1 tablespoon chopped cilantro
2 garlic cloves, peeled and crushed
1 1/2 tablespoons olive oil
2 tablespoons lemon juice
Sprinkle salt
1/4 teaspoon black pepper
1/8 teaspoon cayenne pepper

Peel and boil potatoes. Dice when done. Place diced potatoes in a bowl. Stir in cilantro. Blend remaining ingredients in a blender for only one minute.

Pour mixture over potatoes and serve.

APPENDIX

Essential Fatty Acids

*Linoleic Acid (mg/100 gm)**			
haddock	2.2	coconut oil	2000
sole	7.9	egg yolk	2100
fruits	20	cocoa butter	2100
yogurt	49	olives	2200
venison	120	spices	2400
cream	130	oats	2600
cow's milk	140	butter	2700
goat's milk	200	cashews	3200
spinach	200	wheat germ	4400
lima bealls	220	linseed oil	8000
salmon	230	hazelnuts	9300
cow's meat	240	olive oil	10000
human milk	270	lard	10000
veal	290	almonds	11000
herring	390	peanuts	12000
beans	450	pecans	14000
corn	520	sesame seeds	20000
barley	620	margarine	22000
rice	660	brazil nuts	23000
eggs	780	peanut oil	25000
cheeses	850	walnuts	29000
lamb	1000	sunflower seeds	30000
rye	1200	cottonseed oil	35000
tuna	1200	sesame oil	42000
chicken	1200	wheat germ oil	44000
wheat	1200	walnut oil	48000
turkey	1300	soy oil	52000
soybeans	1400	corn oil	54000
liver	1500	sunflower oil	60000
avocados	1900	canola oil	72000
pig's meat	2000	safflower oil	77000

* Milligrams per 100 grams of food.

Oleic Acid (mg/100 gm)			
lima beans	45	lamb	7100
fruits	100	avocados	7400
spinach	120	olives	7600
beans	120	coconut oil	8600
barley	200	pig's meat	9000
wheat	210	cheeses	9500
rye	280	sesame seeds	10000
corn	340	sunflower oil	12000
rice	660	wheat germ oil	16000
millet	670	cow's meat	18000
human milk	1100	safflower oil	20000
cow's milk	1200	walnuts	21000
tuna	1200	sesame oil	21000
chicken	1200	brazil nuts	21000
egg yolk	1200	peanuts	26000
cream	1300	butter	27000
wheat germ	1500	soy oil	27000
spices	1800	cottonseed oil	30000
oats	2200	cashews	34000
turkey	2600	corn oil	35000
coconut	3100	almonds	37000
haddock	3500	cocoa butter	38000
salmon	4200	pecans	44000
veal	4700	lard	46000
soybeans	4900	hazelnuts	50000
flax seeds	5100	peanut oil	64000
eggs	6000	almond oil	69000
sunflower seeds	6000	olive oil	76000

Minerals

Calcium (mg/100 gm)			
water	0.15	eggs	54
watermelon	3.2	peanuts	69
coffee	3.9	peas	70
plums	4.4	wheat germ	72
honey	4.7	pecans	73
beer	5.0	endive	81
apples	5.3	spinach	93
bananas	5.7	oysters	94
mushrooms	6.1	walnuts	99
whiskey	8.0	chard	100
tuna	8.3	cream	100
wine	8.8	maple syrup	100
egg white	9.0	buckwheat	110
pig's meat	10	cow's milk	120
fruits	10	sunflower seeds	120
avocados	10	kale	130
lamb	11	lentils	130
liver	11	pistachios	130
cow's meat	12	beans	130
tomatoes	12	egg yolk	130
chicken	12	greens	150
coconut	13	chickpeas	150
potatoes	14	salmon	150
cantaloupe	14	watercress	150
cucumber	16	brazil nuts	190
millet	20	parsley	200
butter	20	torula yeast	220
flounder	22	almonds	230
corn	22	soybeans	230
turkey	23	caviar	280
oranges	30	medium molasses	290
vegetables	30	carob	350
rice	32	sardines	350
blackberries	32	brewers yeast	420
human milk	33	sea salt	670
barley	34	cheeses	700
sprouts	35	kelp	1100
wheat	36	sesame seeds	1200
cashews	38	soil	1400
rye	38	seaweed	1900
sea water	40	dolomite	21000
cabbage	49	bone meal (hydroxyapatite)	40000
oats	53		

Most is absorbed.

Chromium (mg/100 gm)			
sea water	0.0000050	maple syrup	0.018
sea salt	0.0000800	grains	0.020
water	0.00018	nuts	0.020
milk	0.00100	butter	0.021
fruits	0.0020	parsley	0.021
carrots	0.0033	blackstrap molasses	0.022
corn	0.0050	chicken	0.026
lard	0.0070	honey	0.029
cow's meat	0.0090	fruits	0.030
vegetable oils	0.0100	vegetables	0.040
pig's meat	0.010	corn oil	0 047
seafood	0.011	brewer's yeast	0.063
lamb	0.012	seaweed	0.130
parsnips	0.013	cloves	0.15
tomatoes	0.014	wheat	0.18
meats	0.014	black pepper	0.37
corn syrup	0.015	thyme	1.00
rice	0.016	soil	10
eggs	0.017		

Less than 1% is absorbed.

Copper (mg/100 gm)			
sea water	0.00030	kale	0.30
water	0.00100	eggplant	0.30
sea salt	0.0047	bee pollen	0.32
tea	0.0100	rice	0.36
coffee	0.020	coconut	0.39
egg white	0.020	avocado	0.39
butter	0.030	tuna	0.50
vegetable oils	0.030	bananas	0.51
egg yolk	0.030	seaweed	0.60
grapefruit	0.040	almonds	0.68
cantaloupe	0.040	barley	0.70
peaches	0.050	lentils	0.71
whiskey	0.060	oats	0.74
eggs	0.070	ginseng	0.75
beer	0 070	cashews	0.76
cow's meat	0.080	salmon	0.80
lettuce	0.090	kelp	0.80
pig's meat	0.090	cloves	0.87
wine	0.100	walnuts	0 90
tomatoes	0.11	brazil nuts	1.1
soybeans	0.11	medium molasses	1.2
vegetables	0.12	hazelnuts	1.4
cheeses	0.14	honey	1.7
dill	0.14	soil	2.0
corn	0.15	black pepper	2.1
cow's milk	0.15	lobster	2.2
potatoes	0.16	blackstrap molasses	2.2
cream	0.17	thyme	2.4
turkey	0.18	wheat germ	2.9
halibut	0.19	mussels	3.2
raw milk	0.19	oysters	3.4
lamb	0.24	liver	3.7
chicken	0.28	mushrooms	6.0

Roughly 45% is absorbed.

Iodine (mg/100 gm)			
water, oranges, and mushrooms	0.00020	cream	0.0060
wine	0.00100	cow's milk	0.0070
whiskey	0.0010	spinach	0.0090
grapefruit	0.0010	eggs	0.0090
beer	0.0010	butter	0.0090
corn	0.0011	lard	0.0097
tomatoes	0.0012	pig's meat	0.0100
wheat	0.0012	lettuce	0.010
green peppers	0.0014	cheeses	0.011
oats	0.0015	potatoes	0.015
beets	0.0016	pineapple	0.016
honey	0.0018	tea	0.016
radishes	0.0018	soybeans	0.017
fruits	0.0020	liver	0.019
almonds	0.0020	cantaloupe	0.020
wheat germ	0:0020	peanuts	0.020
coconut	0.0020	vegetable oils	0.024
tuna	0.0023	crab	0.031
veal	0.0028	halibut	0.046
alfalfa	0.0028	turnip greens	0.047
cashews	0.0030	oysters	0.048
vegetables	0.0030	herring	0.052
walnuts	0.0030	sunflower seeds	0.070
freshwater fishes	0.0030	perch	0.074
lamb	0.0030	sea salt	0.095
apples	0.0030	beans	0.100
salmon	0.0037	lobster	0.10
coffee	0.0040	chard	0.10
medium molasses	0.0040	shrimp	0.13
grains	0.0040	cod	0.14
cow's meat	0.0060	haddock	0.31
peaches	0.0060	soil	0.60
chicken	0.0060	cod liver oil	0.84
sea water	0.0060	iodized salt (U.S.)	10
turkey	0.0060	seaweed	62
		kelp	180

Virtually all is absorbed.

Iron (mg/100 gm)			
butter, cream	0.00	pig's meat	2.9
sea water	0.0010	spinach	3.1
sea salt	0.016	buckwheat	3.1
oranges	0.028	cow's meat	3.1
cow's milk	0.041	veal	3.2
human milk	0.050	brazil nuts	3.4
water	0.067	wheat	3.5
coffee	0.087	snails	3.5
plums	0.19	rye	3.7
egg white	0.20	cashews	3.8
grapefruit	0.21	clams	4.1
watermelon	0.23	oats	4.5
cabbage	0.38	almonds	4.7
wine	0.39	parsley	5.0
fruits	0.40	oysters	5.6
mushrooms	0.49	mussels	5.8
avocado	0.58	walnuts	6.0
honey	0.75	medium molasses	6.0
halibut	0.80	lentils	6.7
cheeses	0.80	millet	6.8
vegetables	1.00	chickpeas	6.9
berries	1.0	sunflower seeds	7.1
potatoes	1.1	mature sprouts	7.2
maple syrup	1.2	egg yolk	7.2
sprouts	1.2	pistachios	7.2
tuna	1.3	liver	8.8
salmon	1.4	blackstrap molasses	9.1
rice	1.6	wheat germ	9.4
bee pollen	1.6	sesame seeds	10
coconut	1.7	pumpkin seeds	11
peas	1.7	caviar	12
chicken	1.8	soy lecithin	12
turkey	2.1	kidney	13
corn	2.1	brewer's yeast	17
peanuts	2.1	torula yeast	18
eggs	2.2	bone meal	82
pecans	2.4	seaweed	90
beans	2.7	kelp	370
barley	2.7	soil	3800

We absorb about 6% of what's eaten.

Magnesium (mg/100 gm)			
bee pollen	0.24	potatoes	27
water	0.41	tuna	29
vegetable oils	0.70	cheeses	30
butter	2.0	bananas	31
human milk	3.0	avocados	37
coffee	5.0	corn	38
apples	5.0	salmon	40
honey	5.5	coconut	44
tea	8.0	barley	55
wine	8.0	spinach	57
pineapple	8.0	chard	65
grapefruit	9.0	mushrooms	68
cream	10	medium molasses	81
egg white	10	rice	120
beer	10	sea water	130
oranges	11	walnuts	130
lettuce	11	oats	140
eggs	12	pecans	140
cow's milk	13	hazelnuts	150
tomatoes	13	soy lecithin	160
fruits	15	pistachios	160
cabbage	15	bone meal	170
egg yolk	16	seaweed	210
oysters	17	brazil nuts	220
carrots	18	soybeans	240
chicken	19	snails	250
lamb	22	almonds	270
liver	22	wheat germ	320
cow's meat	23	sunflower seeds	350
pig's meat	23	blackstrap molasses	410
halibut	23	soil	500
vegetables	25	kelp	740
turkey	25	sea salt	2100
cashews	27	dolomite	13000

About 50% is absorbed.

Manganese (mg/100 gm)			
sea water	0.0002	bone meal	0.50
water	0.0012	kale	0.50
sea salt	0.0032	yams	0.52
cow's meat	0.0050	brewer's yeast	0.53
leeks	0.0100	berries	0.55
cow's milk	0.019	carrots	0.60
chicken	0.020	bananas	0.64
watermelon	0.020	tea	0.69
oranges	0.025	lettuce	0.80.
turkey	0.030	grapefruit	0.80
veal	0.030	spinach	0.82
lemons	0.040	parsley	0 94
cantaloupe	0.040	pineapple	1.1
butter	0.040	coconut	1.3
egg white	0.043	honey	1.4
eggs	0.053	peanuts	1.5
strawberries	0.060	snails	1.6
pig's meat	0.060	rice	1.7
pears	0.060	walnuts	1.8
apples	0.070	turnip greens	1.8
mushrooms	0.080	almonds	1.9
grapes	0.083	beans	2.0
egg yolk	0.088	peas	2.0
lard	0.098	watercress	2.0
fruits	0.100	ginseng	2.0
eggplant	0.11	coffee beans	2.1
kelp	0.15	sunflower seeds	2.5
cucumbers	0.15	brazil nuts	2.8
celery	0.16	barley	3.2
potatoes	0.17	pecans	3.5
cauliflower	0.17	wheat	3.6
vegetable oils	0.18	chestnuts	3.7
tomatoes	0.19	hazelnuts	4.2
apricots	0.20	oats	4.9
fishes	0.20	buckwheat	5.1
liver	0.28	bay leaves	6.7
raspberries	0.28	ginger	8.7
vegetables	0.30	cloves	26
cranberries	0.30	tea leaves	28
blackstrap molasses	0.36	soil	85
rhubarb	0.40	seaweed	120
green beans	0.45		

Roughly 9% is absorbed.

Molybdenum (mg/100 gm)			
water	0.000035	wheat germ	0.056
sea water	0.0010	squash	0.065
seafoods	0.0010	gooseberries	0.068
milk	0.0020	wheat	0.079
haddock	0.0030	rye	0.090
tomatoes	0.0060	dill	0.110
wine	0.0065	liver	0.15
cow's meat	0.0070	soil	0.20
fruits	0.0100	honey	0.20
egg whites	0.012	pig's meat	0.37
chicken	0.014	peas	0.60
sea salt	0.016	beans	0.70
raw milk	0.020	soybeans	1.10
blackstrap molasses	0.029	seaweed	1.6
vegetables	0.050		

Roughly half is absorbed.

Phosphorus (mg/100 gm)			
water	0.0005	pig's meat	230
sea water	0.0070	veal	230
sea salt	0.11	halibut	250
bee pollen	0.40	corn	270
honey	3.1	buckwheat	280
coffee	4.0	pecans	290
plums	6.2	chicken	290
maple syrup	8.0	barley	290
apples	10	millet	310
whisky	10	turkey	320
wine	10	chickpeas	330
human milk	14	kelp	340
egg white	16	flounder	340
butter	16	mature sprouts	340
cucumber	18	tuna	350
tea	19	scallops	360
fruits	20	cashews	370
lettuce	22	wheat	380
tomatoes	27	lentils	380
beer	30	rye	380
light molasses	36	salmon	400
vegetables	40	peas	400
avocados	42	beans	400
soil	65	peanuts	400
mushrooms	68	oats	410
medium molasses	69	liver	480
sprouts	70	almonds	500
cream	80	soybeans	550
carob	80	walnuts	570
blackstrap molasses	85	egg yolk	570
cow's milk	93	sardines	580
coconut	95	pine nuts	600
radishes	100	sesame seeds	620
parsley	100	brazil nuts	690
kale	110	sunflower seeds	840
oysters	120	wheat germ	1100
cow's meat	190	pumpkin seeds	1100
eggs	200	torula yeast	1500
seaweed	210	brewer's yeast	1800
lamb	210	soy lecithin	3300
rice	220	dolomite	26000

Most is absorbed.

Potassium (mg/100 gm)			
water	0.23	sprouts	320
whiskey	2.0	oats	350
yogurt	20	bananas	370
butter	23	cow's meat	370
beer	25	liver	380
tea	25	wheat	390
peaches	27	potatoes	410
coffee	36	chicken	430
sea water	38	millet	430
human milk	50	turkey	440
honey	51	buckwheat	450
plums	63	cashews	460
watermelon	65	walnuts	460
oysters	70	rye	470
concord grapes	78	salmon	510
cheeses	80	halibut	530
wine	80	veal	580
pears	100	lentils	590
grapefruit	110	avocados	600
apples	110	pecans	600
cream	110	soil	630
egg yolk	120	peanuts	670
eggs	130	brazil nuts	720
onions	140	sesame seeds	720
cow's milk	140	almonds	770
green grapes	150	chickpeas	800
berries	150	sunflower seeds	920
egg white	150	wheat germ	950
cucumber	160	pistachios	980
oranges	170	mature sprouts	1000
maple syrup	180	sea salt	1000
tuna	180	peas	1000
fruits	200	parsley	1000
rice	210	medium molasses	1100
cabbage	230	beans	1200
cantaloupe	250	blackstrap molasses	1700
coconut	260	soybeans	1700
corn	280	brewer's yeast	1900
pig's meat	290	torula yeast	2000
lamb	300	seaweed	5200
vegetables	300	kelp	12000

About 90% is absorbed.

Selenium (mg/100 gm)			
sea water	0.000040	peanuts	0.038
apples	0.000500	alfalfa	0.038
cream	0.00050	rice	0.039
green beans	0.00060	seaweed	0.043
sea salt	0.00064	liver	0.050
bananas	0.00100	freshwater fishes	0.050
cow's milk	0.0012	saltwater fishes	0.053
human milk	0.0021	soybeans	0.054
carrots	0.0022	shellfish	0.060
beans	0.0030	tomatoes	0.060
torula yeast	0.0040	barley	0.062
cheeses	0.0080	beets	0.065
egg	0.0100	chicken	0.070
brewer's yeast	0.011	onions	0.080
lentils	0.011	vegetable oils	0.100
oats	0.012	peas	0.12
grains	0.015	beans	0.12
egg yolk	0.018	wheat	0.13
rye	0.020	mushrooms	0.14
soil	0.020	cabbage	0.25
garlic	0.020	corn	0.40
meats	0.022		

60% is absorbed.

Sodium (mg/100 gm)			
salt	39000	cabbage	20
sea salt	30000	human milk	17
kelp	4000	light molasses	15
seaweed	3300	torula yeast	15
sea water	1900	cashews	15
soil	1400	vegetables	10
egg white	190	maple syrup	10
brewer's yeast	120	rice	9.0
eggs	120	beer	7.0
shellfish	100	beans	7.0
oyster	94	unsalted butter	7 0
blackstrap molasses	91	walnuts	6.0
veal	82	wine	5.0
flounder	78	barley	5 0
celery	75	honey	5.0
sablefish	73	soybeans	5.0
spinach	71	peanuts	5.0
lamb	70	potatoes	4.2
liver	70	almonds	4.0
turkey	62	avocados	4.0
cow's meat	60	scallions	4.0
sesame seeds	60	tomatoes	3.0
pig's meat	57	wheat	2.3
egg yolk	53	oats	1.4
fishes	50	clams	1.2
carrots	50	sprouts	1.2
watercress	50	fruits	1.0
yogurt	47	brazil nuts	1.0
cow's milk	47	whiskey	1.0
salmon	45	rye	1.0
cream	43	buckwheat	0.91
medium molasses	37	coffee	0.90
tuna	37	corn	0.80
peas	35	water	0.63
sunflower seeds	30	tea	0.43
lentils	30	pecans	0.29
chickpeas	26	watermelon	0.22
parsley	25	millet	0.20
coconut	23		

Most is absorbed.

Vanadium (mg/100 gm)			
cow's milk	0.0000010	ginseng	0.0023
apples	0.0000027	sea salt	0.0032
cauliflower	0.0000076	lobster	0.0043
tomatoes	0.0000078	radishes	0.0052
fruits	0.0000400	meats	0.0100
potatoes	0.000082	dill	0.014
water	0.000100	nuts	0.070
human milk	0.00018	parsley	0.079
sea water	0.00020	grains	0.110
calf's liver	0.00024	seafood	0.17
mackerel	0.00026	vegetable oils	0.34
sardines	0.00090	seaweed	0.53
lettuce	0.00210		

0.640% of eaten vanadium is absorbed.

Zinc (mg/100 gm)			
sea water	0.0010	almonds	1.5
water	0.0010	rice	1.5
sea salt	0.016	millet	1.5
greens	0.070	mangoes	1.9
peaches	0.090	clams	2.0
wine	0.100	buckwheat	2.0
grapefruit	0.10	eggs	2.1
whiskey	0.10	bleu cheese	2.2
cantaloupe	0.10	peas	2.3
beer	0.10	avocados	2.4
lettuce	0.10	beans	2.4
oranges	0.10	barley	2.7
apples	0.10	walnuts	2.8
fruits	0.12	turkey	2.8
cherries	0.15	beets	2.8
radishes	0.16	cow's meat	3.0
squash	0.21	coconut	3.0
cauliflower	0.23	corn	3.1
tomatoes	0.24	wheat	3.2
pineapple	0.26	rye	3.4
bananas	0.28	pig's meat	3.4
cream	0.30	seaweed	3.5
butter	0.30	bone meal	3.6
egg white	0.30	oats	3.7
vegetable oils	0.32	brewer's yeast	3.9
vegetables	0.35	medium molasses	4.6
milk	0.40	cocoa	4.8
mushrooms	0.40	chicken	4.8
tuna	0.50	soil	5.0
carrots	0.50	lamb	5.4
lard	0.50	egg yolk	5.5
spinach	0.70	sunflower seeds	6.6
cabbage	0.80	soybeans	6.7
kale	0.82	liver	7.0
cheeses	0.90	maple syrup	7.5
honey	0.90	blackstrap molasses	8.3
parsley	0.90	torula yeast	9.9
halibut	1.00	sesame seeds	10
cashews	1.0	wheat germ	14
bran	1.1	herring	110
turnips	1.2	oysters	160
salmon	1.4		

About 40% is absorbed.

Vitamins

Vitamin A (International Units/100 gm)

Food	IU	Food	IU
mushrooms	0	salmon	300
egg white	0	walnuts	300
white grapefruit	10	plums	300
sprouts	15	oysters	310
pears	20	summer squash	400
beets	20	green peppers	420
sesame seeds	30	tangerines	420
sardines	30	pink grapefruit	440
olives	33	mackerel	450
pine nuts	38	okra	520
sunflower seeds	50	mature sprouts	550
shrimp	50	watermelon	590
chickpeas	50	kumquats	600
lentils	58	soybeans	700
cauliflower	60	halibut	850
strawberries	60	asparagus	900
bluefish	62	tomatoes	900
yogurt	70	lobster	920
pineapple	70	cream	1000
tuna	80	lettuce	1000
apples	90	cherries	1000
rhubarb	100	eggs	1200
blueberries	100	cheeses	1300
cashews	100	peaches	1300
grapes	100	pitangas	1500
bass	100	pumpkin	1600
soy lecithin	100	eel	1600
clams	100	nectarines	1600
hazelnuts	110	papayas	1700
cow's milk	125	mangoes	1800
raspberries	130	romaine	1900
pecans	130	whitefish	2000
cabbage	130	swordfish	2100
avocados	150	crab	2200
artichoke	150	pimentoes	2300
herring	150	broccoli	2500
cod	170	apricots	2700
oranges	200	persimmons	2700
pistachios	230	endive	3300
human milk	240	cantaloupe	3400
cucumbers	250	egg yolk	3400
guavas	280	winter squash	4000

B^1 — *Thiamin (mg/100 gm)*

whiskey, wine, tea, corn syrup, coffee, honey and soda	0.00
human milk	0.01
soy lecithin	0.01
goat's milk	0.01
egg white	0.01
cow's milk	0:03
cheeses	0.03
fruits	0.03
radishes	0.03
shrimp	0.03
sardines	0 03
skim milk	0 04
yogurt	0.04
onions	0 04
cucumbers	0.04
tuna	0.05
coconut	0.05
Barbados molasses	0.06
chicken	0.06
light molasses	0.07
oranges	0 07
vegetables	0.08
cow's meat	0.08
medium molasses	0.09
pineapple	0.09
mushrooms	0.10
clams	0.10
avocado	0.11
turkey	0.11
potatoes	0.11
veal	0.13
oysters	0.14
mackerel	0.15
lamb	0.15
eggs	0.17
sprouts	0.18
salmon	0.21
barley	0.21
almonds	0.24
liver	0.25
blackstrap molasses	0.28
chickpeas	0.31
egg yolk	0.32
walnuts	0.33
rice	0 34
corn	0 37
lentils	0.37
mature sprouts	0.40
rye	0.43
hazelnuts	0.46
eel	0.50
wheat	0 57
oats	0.60
buckwheat	0.60
beans	0.68
pig's meat	0.70
millet	0.73
peas	0.80
alfalfa	0.80
pecans	0.86
bee pollen	0.93
brazil nuts	0.96
sesame seeds	0.98
soybeans	1.10

B^2 — Riboflavin (mg/100 gm)

gelatin, oils	0.00
wine	0.01
fruits	0.02
watercress	0.02
coconut	0.02
shrimp	0.03
celery	0.03
beer	0.03
soy lecithin	0.03
honey	0.04
tomatoes	0.04
mayonnaise	0.04
onions	0.04
papaya	0.04
peaches	0.04
cabbage	0.04
rice	0.05
carrots	0.05
herring	0.05
lettuce	0.05
light molasses	0.06
strawberries	0.07
barley	0.07
raspberries	0.09
goat's milk	0.11
brazil nuts	0.12
medium molasses	0.12
vegetables	0.12
fishes	0.12
wheat	0.12
peanuts	0.13
walnuts	0.13
pecans	0.13
oats	0.14
cream cheese	0.15
chickpeas	0.15
buckwheat	0.17
cow's milk	0.17
yogurt	0.18
clams	0.18
sprouts	0.19
corn	0.19
raw milk	0.19
cow's meat	0.20
broccoli	0.20
pig's meat	0.20
Barbados molasses	0.20
turkey	0.20
spinach	0.20
beans	0.22
rye	0.22
lentils	0.22
egg white	0.22
sesame seeds	0.24
cottage cheese	0.25
parsley	0.25
blackstrap molasses	0.25
peas	0.25
lamb	0.27
sunflower seeds	0.28
eggs	0.28
veal	0.31
soybeans	0.31
mushrooms	0.33
chicken	0.36
millet	0.38
human milk	0.40
cheeses	0.46
egg yolk	0.52
mustard greens	0.64
wheat germ	0.68
almonds	0.92
bee pollen	1.7
alfalfa	1.8
royal jelly	1.9
liver	4.1
brewer's yeast	4.2
torula yeast	16

B^3 — Niacin (mg/100 gm)			
sugar	0.00	brazil nuts	1.6
mayonnaise	0.01	cashews	1.8
soy lecithin	0.01	chickpeas	2.0
cream	0.04	lentils	2.0
apples	0.07	blackstrap molasses	2.1
chard	0.07	corn	2.2
watermelon	0.08	soybeans	2.2
grapefruit	0.08	millet	2.3
yogurt	0.08	beans	2.4
milk	0.08	oysters	2.5
pecans	0.09	mature sprouts	2.6
tangerines	0.09	peas	2.6
cheeses	0.10	shrimp	3.3
egg white	0.10	almonds	3.5
wine	0.10	barley	3.7
plums	0.19	wheat germ	4.2
cucumbers	0.20	mushrooms	4.2
eggs	0.20	wheat	4.3
grapes	0.20	buckwheat	4.3
human milk	0.20	pine nuts	4.5
light molasses	0.20	wheat bran	4.7
celery	0.25	rice	4.7
radishes	0.25	potatoes	4.8
coffee	0.26	alfalfa	5.0
cabbage	0.28	cow's meat	5.0
goat's milk	0.30	sesame seeds	5.4
coconut	0.44	sardines	5.4
honey	0.48	pig's meat	5.5
fruits	0.60	sunflower seeds	5.6
beer	0.61	veal	7.8
vegetables	0.65	royal jelly	8.2
walnuts	0.71	halibut	9.2
sprouts	0.80	rabbit	11
peaches	0.87	turkey	11
raspberries	0.89	swordfish	11
hazelnuts	0.90	tuna	12
oats	1.00	chicken	12
bleu cheese	1.2	salmon	13
medium molasses	1.2	liver	16
clams	1.3	peanuts	17
collard greens	1.3	bee pollen	19
avocado	1.6	brewer's yeast	38
rye	1.6	torula yeast	100

B^5 — Pantothenic Acid (mg/100 gm)			
soy lecithin	0.05	perch	0.80
beer	0.10	walnuts	0.90
egg white	0.14	turkey	0.90
oysters	0.20	sardines	0.90
fruits	0.20	chicken	0.90
honey	0.20	mushrooms	1.00
coconut	0.20	avocado	1.1
cream	0.20	chickpeas	1.2
brazil nuts	0.23	cashews	1.3
blackberries	0.25	lobster	1.5
blackstrap molasses	0.30	bleu cheese	1.8
vegetables	0.30	wheat germ	2.2
milk	0.30	bee pollen	2.2
shrimp	0.30	eggs	2.3
halibut	0.30	rye	2.6
clams	0.30	peanuts	2.8
bran	0.35	wheat	3.2
beans	0.40	alfalfa	3.3
skim milk	0.40	peas	3.6
almonds	0.50	egg yolk	4.2
cheeses	0.50	lentils	4.8
broccoli	0 50	corn	5.0
cow's meat	0.50	soybeans	5.2
barley	0.50	sunflower seeds	5.5
tuna	0.50	rice	8.9
potatoes	0.50	torula yeast	10
pig's meat	0.50	brewer's yeast	11
lamb	0.60	royal jelly	35
salmon	0.80		

B^6 — Pyridoxine (mg/100 gm)

Food	mg/100 gm	Food	mg/100 gm
butter	0.000	pig's meat	0.32
coffee	0.010	banana	0.32
honey	0.020	lamb	0.32
apples	0.030	halibut	0.34
cream	0.030	cow's meat	0.40
soy lecithin	0.030	chicken	0.40
milk	0.040	oats	0.40
oysters	0.040	turkey	0.40
coconut	0.040	peanuts	0.40
mushrooms	0.050	cashews	0.40
beer	0.060	beans	0.57
fruits	0.070	shrimp	0.60
cheeses	0.080	avocados	0.60
clams	0.080	liver	0.67
almonds	0.100	peas	0.67
vegetables	0.15	walnuts	0.73
brazil nuts	0.17	bran	0.85
bleu cheese	0.17	tuna	0.90
pecans	0.18	wheat germ	0.92
sardines	0.18	salmon	0.98
potatoes	0.20	alfalfa	1.00
medium molasses	0.20	hazelnuts	1.1
barley	0.21	sunflower seeds	1.1
green peppers	0.26	lentils	1.7
eggs	0.27	rye	1.8
mackerel	0.27	soybeans	2.0
spinach	0.28	royal jelly	2.4
egg yolk	0.30	wheat	2.9
corn	0.30	rice	3.6
blackstrap molasses	0.31	brewer's yeast	4.0

B^{12} — Cobalamin (mg/100 gm)

Food	mg/100 gm
vegetables, fruits, oil, nuts and yeast	0.00000000
sunflower seeds	0.00000040
yogurt	0.000060
egg white	0.000090
butter	0.000100
cream cheese	0.00022
buttermilk	0.00022
cream	0.00035
milk	0.00040
turkey	0.00042
cod	0.00050
chicken	0.00050
cottage cheese	0.00059
pig's meat	0.00060
anchovies	0.00062
shrimp	0:00082
crab	0.00085
cheeses	0.00100
scallops	0.0011
egg yolk	0.0012
camembert	0.0012
gorgonzola	0.0012
bass	0.0013
halibut	0.0013
lobster	0.0013
liverwurst	0.0014
sausage	0.0014
bleu cheese	0.0014
cow's meat	0.0015
swordfish	0.0015
muenster cheese	0.0016
haddock	0.0017
puffer	0.0018
eggs	0.0020
swiss cheese	0.0021
octopus	0.0029
lamb	0.0031
salmon	0.0047
hake	0.0049
squid	0.0050
flounder	0.0064
snapper	0.0088
croaker	0.0094
herring	0.0100
mackerel	0.0100
clam broth	0.0100
clams	0.020
sardines	0.034
liver	0.086

Biotin (mg/100 gm)			
soy lecithin	0.00	eggs	0.020
potatoes	0.00010	wheat germ	0.020
apples	0.0010	clams	0.020
human milk	0.0010	mackerel	0.020
fruits	0.0025	corn	0.021
cheeses	0.0036	sardines	0.024
cow's meat	0.0040	oats	0.024
yams	0.0043	wheat	0.027
bananas	0.0044	pecans	0.030
cow's milk	0.0047	cashews	0.030
vegetables	0.0050	tuna	0.030
avocados	0.0060	alfalfa	0.030
pig's meat	0.0062	barley	0.031
goat's milk	0.0063	chickpeas	0.032
egg white	0.0070	peanuts	0.040
sprouts	0.0080	walnuts	0.040
halibut	0.0080	lentils	0.042
oysters	0.0087	green peas	0.042
shrimp	0.010	egg yolk	0.052
turkey	0.010	rice germ	0.058
medium molasses	0.010	rice bran	0.060
lamb	0.010	rice	0.070
coconut	0.010	sunflower seeds	0.070
chicken	0.011	split peas	0.082
bran	0.014	butter	0.100
salmon	0.015	torula yeast	0.10
mushrooms	0.016	liver	0.12
cauliflower	0.017	soybeans	0.19
beans	0.017	brewer's yeast	0.20
almonds	0.018	royal jelly	0.29
bee pollen	0.020	rye	0.33
blackstrap molasses	0.020		

Choline (mg/100 gm)			
apples	1.0	bran	140
egg white	2.0	alfalfa	140
vegetable oils	5.0	blackstrap molasses	150
fruits	10	sprouts	210
yams	12	sunflower seeds	220
milk	15	brewer's yeast	240
cheeses	50	peanuts	240
pecans	50	spinach	240
cow's meat	70	torula yeast	250
corn	71	cabbage	250
trout	87	green peas	270
wheat	92	green beans	340
corn	92	soybeans	340
oats	94	wheat germ	400
carrots	95	eggs	500
vegetables	100	caviar	540
veal	100	liver	550
potatoes	110	rice	650
flax seeds	110	split peas	700
lamb	110	lentils	710
pig's meat	120	chickpeas	780
asparagus	130	egg yolk	1700
barley	140	soy lecithin	2900

Folacin (mg/100 gm)			
tuna	0.0010	almonds	0.050
egg white	0.0010	brazil nuts	0.050
shrimp	0.0020	broccoli	0.050
lamb	0.0030	brussels sprouts	0.050
clams	0.0030	corn	0.059
pig's meat	0.0030	greens	0.060
carrots	0.0080	walnuts	0.060
human milk	0.0100	soy lecithin	0.060
medium molasses	0.010	peanuts	0.060
potatoes	0.010	kale	0 070
radishes	0.010	hazelnuts	0.070
turkey	0.010	spinach	0.080
green peppers	0.010	collard greens	0.100
cheeses	0.010	sunflower seeds	0.10
fruits	0.010	green peas	0.11
salmon	0.011	asparagus	0.12
cow's milk	0.011	sprouts	0.14
egg yolk	0.013	rice	0.17
vegetables	0.020	barley	0.21
mushrooms	0.020	wheat	0.22
halibut	0.020	split peas	0.23
cream	0.020	liver	0.29
cashews	0.025	wheat germ	0.31
bananas	0.030	beans	0.31
coconut	0.030	lentils	0.34
eggs	0.030	oats	0.39
sardines	0.030	chickpeas	0.41
cottage cheese	0.030	endive	0.47
pecans	0 030	soybeans	0.69
rye	0.035	alfalfa	0.80
bran	0.040	brewer's yeast	2.0
cow's meat	0.040	torula yeast	3.0

Inositol (mg/100 gm)			
halibut	17	cantaloupe	120
salmon	18	strawberries	120
eggs	22	sunflower seed	150
cheeses	25	grapefruit	150
potatoes	29	peas	160
vegetables	30	wheat	170
apples	31	blackstrap molasses	170
oysters	44	peanuts	180
turnip greens	46	alfalfa	210
chicken	48	oranges	210
carrots	48	beans	240
tomatoes	50	cow's meat	260
corn	50	torula yeast	270
cow's milk	50	oats	320
brewer's yeast	50	liver	340
lettuce	55	veal	340
lamb	57	barley	390
watermelon	64	pig's meat	410
yams	66	lentils	410
sprouts	70	wheat germ	690
fruits	80	rice	700
human milk	92	chickpeas	760
cabbage	95	tea leaves	1000
cauliflower	95	soy lecithin	2100

Vitamin C (mg/100 gm)	
beans, dairy, nuts, grain and meat	0.0
plums	1.9
tamarinds	2.0
lettuce	2.4
pomegranates	3.0
watermelon	3.2
grapes	3.6
apples	4 0
pears	4.0
peaches	6.1
casaba melon	7.0
carrots	8.0
cherries	8.7
rhubarb	9.0
pumpkin	9.0
persimmons, Jap.	9.0
mammee fruit	9.0
apricots	10
cranberries	10
bananas	10
endive	10
onions	10
cucumbers	11
mulberries	12
nectarines	13
blueberries	14
sapodillos	14
avocados	14
quinces	15
horevdew melon	15
royal jelly	16
tangelos	16
pineapple	17
romaine lettuce	18
raspberries	18
squash	22
tomatoes	23
tangerines	23
loganberries	24
radosjes	24
lychees	25
pitangas	25
mangoes	27
breadfruit	29
limes	31
green onions	32
cantaloupe	33
lemons	35
dandelion greens	35
kumquats	36
elderberries	36
papaya	37
grapefruit	38
cabbage	47
oranges	50
spinach	51
persimmons, native	52
strawberries	57
chives	70
amaranths	80
watercress	80
green peppers	110
parsley	170
black currants	200
guavas	240
acerola cherries	1100
rose hips	3000

Vitamin D (IU/100 gm)			
egg white	0.0	eggs	48
bass	1.0	liver	50
bee pollen	1.6	sunflower seeds	92
cow's milk	4.0	shrimp	150
cottage cheese	4.0	mushrooms	150
human milk	6.0	egg yolk	160
corn oil	9.0	tuna	250
oysters	10	salmon	400
cream	15	sardines	500
cheeses	30	cod liver oil	20,000
butter	40	tuna liver oil	10,000,000

Vitamin E (IU/100 gm)	
mushrooms	0.0
skim milk	0.0
cow's milk	0.060
cottage cheese	0.100
lamb	0.20
pig's meat	0.20
beans	0.20
cow's meat	0.20
medium molassas	0.20
chicken	0.20
human milk	0.23
fruits	0.30
vegetables	0.30
turkey	0.30
yeast	0.40
carrots	0.50
shrimp	0 50
halibut	0.60
apples	0.60
liver	0.60
coconut oil	0.60
cream	0 70
coconut	1.00
leeks	1.0
eggs	1.0
cheeses	1.0
lard	1.0
rye	1.2
bee pollen	1.3
salmon	1.4
pecans	1.5
avocados	1.5
corn	1.7
barley	1.7
oats	1.7
parsley	1.8
butter	1.9
broccoli	2.0
vegetable oils	2.3
asparagus	2.6
spinach	2.9
soy lecithin	4.8
cashews	5.1
cod liver oil	5.4
peanuts	6.5
brazil nuts	6.5
almond oil	7.5
cabbage	7.8
mayonnaise	12
margarine	13
olive oil	14
almonds	15
peanut oil	16
soy oil	16
apricot oil	21
hazelnuts	21
corn oil	21
walnuts	22
sesame oil	26
wheat	30
sunflower seeds	31
safflower oil	35
cottonseed oil	44
wheat germ	160

Vitamin K (mg/100 gm)			
oranges	0.0011	coffee	0.039
eggs	0.0020	peas	0.044
cauliflower	0.0020	watercress	0.060
bananas	0.0020	bran	0.069
cow's milk	0.0029	potatoes	0.080
green beans	0 0044	liver	0.100
corn oil	0.0071	broccoli	0.20
peaches	0.0079	cabbage	0.25
mushrooms	0.0083	cauliflower	0.28
asparagus	0.0100	soybeans	0.30
corn	0.010	spinach	0.33
carrots	0.010	oats	0.49
eggs	0.012	alfalfa	0.52
strawberries	0.013	pig's meat	0.95
honey	0.025	soy lecithin	1.2
tomatoes	0.027	brussel sprouts	1.5
wheat germ	0.033	camembert	16.0
cow's meat	0.035	cheddar	22.0

A List of Foods With Generally Recognized Strengthening or Aphrodisiac Properties

asparagus
peas
lentils
beans (kidney)
haricot beans
artichokes
spinach
onions (french, spanish, egyptian)
garlic
horseradish

radishes
beetroot
tarragon
coriander
mint
gentian
saffron
thyme
cloves
sage
marjoram

ginger
cinnamon
nutmeg
cardamom
red pepper
white pepper
cubeb pepper
paprika
curry powder
kola

various aromatic spices
crab
lobster
crayfish
shrimps
oysters
mussels
cockles
clams
herring
salmon
mackerel
plaice
whiting
cod liver
cod liver oil
halibut
halibut liver oil
soft herring roe
cod roe
caviar
mutton and lamb
beef
veal
ham
chicken
goose
duck
pheasant
hare
liver (various)

animal testes
kidneys
tripe
glucose
sugar
milk
yeast
marmite
eggs (all kinds)
sauces (various)
banana
peaches
fresh figs
pineapples (cooked with sugar)
cherries
grapes (black and white)
pure grape juice
tomatoes

Bovril
Lemco (made by Oxo)

Sanatogen (and other patent foods such as Bynogen)

special soups (listed under soups in recipes)

beer
burgundy
Abricotine (apricot brandy dist. in France)
Absinthe (Pernod Fils is the best)
cider
arrack (an eastern spirit flavored with fruits and herbs)
Chateau d'Yquem (sauternes)
Vouvray (a white wine – French)
Champagne
tawny port (small quantities)
white port
Tarragona
Saumur (white and red)
Sauternes
Prunelle de Bourgogne (liqueur)
flips (eggs and alcohol)
Armagnac
Beaujolais and Barsad

Bibliography

Adams, Ruth, and Frank Murray. *All You Should Know About Health Foods,* Atlanta, GA: Communication Channels, 1983.

—*Body, Mind and the B-Vitamins.* New York: Pinnacle Books, 1975.

—*The Good Seeds, the Rich Grains, the Hardy Nuts for a Healthier, Happier Life.* Atlanta, GA: Communication Channels, 1977.

Airola, Paavo. *Health Secrets from Europe.* New York: Arco Publishing Inc., 1971.

—*How to Get Well.* Scottsdale, AZ: Health Plus Publishers, 1987.

—*The Miracle of Garlic.* Scottsdale, AZ: Health Plus Publishers, 1987.

—*Worldwide Secrets for Staying Young,* Scottsdale, AZ: Health Plus Publishers, 1982.

Atkins, Robert, M.D. *Dr. Atkins' Nutrition Breakthrough: How to Treat Your Medical Condition Without Drugs.* New York: Bantam Books Inc., 1982.

A Barefoot Doctor's Manual: *The American Translation of the Official Chinese Paramedical Manual.* Philadelphia: Running Press Book Publishers, 1977.

Benowicz, Robert J. *Vitamins and You.* New York: Berkley Publishing Group, 1984.

Bey, Pilaff. *Venus in the Kitchen or Love's Cookery Book.* Edited by Norman Douglas. London: William Heinemann Ltd., 1952.

Brillat-Savarin, Anthelme. *Physiology of Taste.* Translated by M.F.K. Fisher. San Diego, CA: Harcourt Brace Jovanovich, 1978.

Brooks, Marvin, and Sally Brooks. *Lifelong Lover.* New York: Doubleday Publishing Co., 1986.

Cheraskin, E., and W.M. Ringsdorff, Jr. *Psychodietetics.* New York: Bantam Books Inc.,1976.

Colbin, Annemarie. *Food and Healing.* New York: Ballantine/Del Rey/Fawcett Books, 1986.

Colgan, Michael. *Your Personal Vitamin Profile: A Medical Scientist Shows You How to Chart Your Individual Vitamin and Mineral Formula.* New York: William Morrow & Co., Inc., 1982.

Culpeper, Nicholas. *Complete Herbal.* Cedar Knolls, NJ: Wehman, 1970.

—*Culpeper's Color Herbal.* New York: Sterling Publishing Co., Inc., 1983.

Cureton, Thomas Kirk. *Physiological Effects of Wheat Germ Oil on Humans in Exercise: Forty-two Physical Training Programs Utilizing 894 Humans.* Springfield, IL: Charles C. Thomas, Publisher, 1972.

Dioscorides, Pedanius. *The Greek Herbal of Dioscorides.* New York: Hafner/Macmillan, 1959.

Fredericks, Carlton. *Carlton Fredericks' Program for Living Longer.* New York: Simon & Schuster Inc., 1983.

—*Food Facts and Fallacies.* New York: Arco Publishing Inc., 1968.

Gottlieb, Adam. *Sex, Drugs and Aphrodisiacs.* San Francisco: 20th Century Alchemist/High Times/Level Press, 1974.

Heffern, Richard. *Complete Book of Ginseng.* Berkeley, CA: Celestial Arts/Ten Speed Press, 1976.

Kugler, Hans J. *Slowing Down the Aging Process.* New York: Pyramid Publications, 1973.

Lesser, Michael, M.D. *Nutrition and Vitamin Therapy.* New York: Bantam Books Inc., 1981.

Lust, John. *The Herb Book.* New York: Bantam Books Inc., 1974.

Mannerberg, Don, M.D., and June Roth. *Aerobic Nutrition.* New York: Berkley Publishing Group, 1983.

Meyer, C. *Herbal Aphrodisiacs.* Glenwood IL: Meyerbooks.

Mindell, Earl. *Earl Mindell's New and Revised Vitamin Bible.* New York: Warner Books Inc., 1985.

—*Shaping Up With Vitamins.* New York: Warner Books Inc., 1985.

Nittler, Alan H., M.D. *A New Breed of Doctor.* New York: Pyramid Publications, 1972.

Ovid, *The Art of Love.* Translated by Rolfe Humphries. Bloomington, IN: Indiana University Press, 1957.

Passwater, Richard A. *Supernutrition.* New York: Pocket Books, 1975.

Pearson, Durk, and Sandy Shaw. *Life Extension.* New York: Warner Books Inc., 1983.

The Perfumed Garden for the Soul's Delectation. Translated from the Arabic of the Shaykh al Nafzawi by Sir Richard F. Burton. London: Spearman, 1981.

Robinson, William J., M.D. *Treatment of Sexual Impotence in Men and Women.* New York: Eugenics Publishing Company, 1931.

Scala, James. *Making the Vitamin Connection.* New York: Harper & Row, Publishers, Inc., 1985.

Steiner, Claude M., Ph.D. *When a Man Loves a Woman: Sexual and Emotional Literacy for the Modern Man.* New York: Grove Press, 1986.

Stekel, Wilhelm. *Impotence in the Male.* New York: Liveright/ W.W. Norton, 1971.

Tierra, Michael. *The Way of Herbs.* New York: Washington Square Press, 1980.

Van de Velde, Theodoor H. *Ideal Marriage: Its Physiology and Technique.* Second Edition. Edited by Margaret Smyth. Westport, CT: Greenwood Press, 1980.

Vatsyayana. *Kama Sutra.* Translated by Sir Richard Burton. Winchester, MA: Allen & Unwin Inc., 1981.

Vaughan, William J. *Low Salt Secrets for Your Diet.* New York: Warner Books Inc., 1984.

Venette, Nicholas. *Conjugal Love: or the Pleasures of the Marriage Bed.* New York: Garland Publishing Inc., 1984.

Wade, Carlson. *Bee Pollen and Your Health.* New Canaan, CT: Keats Publishing Inc., 1978.

—*Carlson Wade's Amino Acids Book.* New Canaan, CT: Keats Publishing Inc., 1985.

—*Health Tonics, Elixirs and Potions for the Look and Feel of Youth.* New York: Arco Publishing Inc., 1973.

—*Lecithin Book.* New Canaan, CT: Keats Publishing Inc., 1980.

—*Vitamins, Minerals and Other Supplements.* New Canaan, CT: Keats Publishing Inc., 1983.

Wedeck, H.E. *Dictionary of Aphrodisiacs.* New York: Philosophical Library.

Williams, Roger J. *Nutrition Against Disease,* White Plains, NY: Pitman/Longman Inc., 1971.

—*A Physician's Handbook on Orthomolecular Medicine.* New Canaan, CT: Keats Publishing Inc., 1979.